6

F Dear Devora,

Best Wishes!

[signature]

Larry North

LIVING LEAN ∎

The

Larry North

Program

A Fireside Book

Published by Simon & Schuster

FIRESIDE
Rockefeller Center
1230 Avenue of the Americas
New York, NY 10020

FIRESIDE and colophon are registered trademarks
of Simon & Schuster Inc.

Designed by Richard Oriolo

Exercise photographs ©1996 by Seth A. Smith.
Photographs on pages 8, 16, 88, 93,100, and 147
©1996 by Hans di Milano—Dallas. Other photographs property of
Larry North or used by permission.

Manufactured in the United States of America

2 3 4 5 6 7 8 9 10

Library of Congress Cataloging-in-Publication Data
North, Larry
Living lean : the Larry North program / Larry North.
p.   cm.
Includes index.
1. Weight loss.   2. Reducing diets.   3. Reducing exercises.
4. Physical fitness.   I. Title.
RA776.5.N68   1997
613.2'5—dc21   96-46973   CIP

ISBN 0-684-83700-5

The instructions and advice in this book are in no way intended as
a substitute for medical counseling. We advise the reader to consult with his/her doctor before beginning this or any regimen of exercise. The author and the publisher disclaim any liability or loss,
personal or otherwise, resulting from the procedures in this book.

To my lovely wife Melanie, my mom, Adam and Alan

Contents

Acknowledgments

I've never before been so excited about acknowledging the people who have helped me over the last several years and led me to the writing of *Living Lean*.

I've known a lot of hardworking people and I'd have to say that my editor, Cindy Gitter, works as hard as anyone I've ever met in my life. That's what made it so difficult ever to refuse one of her many requests.

I want to thank her assistant, Matt Walker, for helping put the book together and for putting up with my thousands of phone calls.

It's one thing to know the world's most knowledgeable nutritionist and another to be able to consider him one of your best friends. Keith Klein's nutritional input to this book was invaluable.

Dr. Joey Antonio, who help substantiate the scientific information in *Living Lean* as well as helping in my radio and television shows, continues to make science fun and interesting.

There are not enough pages in this book to express my gratitude to my wife. Not only did she stay calm while I went insane, she was and has continued to be the spirit, inspiration, and motivation that keeps me going—besides being the one who created every recipe in this book along with the information for the cooking chapter. Mel, I love you.

Larry North Total Fitness is the finest health-club organization in the country mainly because of my CEO and close friend, Steve Mekuly, and partners Jim Prochaska and Karen Tickman. Thank you all for continuing to promote and believe in me.

Special thanks to our assistants Devon Hendry, Cydne Johnson, and Cathy Odom and everyone at the Larry North Total Fitness organization. You are simply the best.

It was unique to have a workout partner who was also writing a book. Skip Bayless, you are an extraordinary man and a great friend who always knows when to push me.

I also want to thank the models who appear in the workout chapter: Paula Deason, Pamela Guyton, Darlyn Grammer, and Angel Cope.

NorthSouth restaurant has been very exciting to be a part of, and my partner, James Cook and all of the staff have been wonderful.

Darwin Deason, who is my partner in NorthSouth, as well as a workout partner and a very close friend, your influence on me is off the charts. Thanks for everything.

I must mention KTCK and KRLD radio with special thanks to Michael Spears. My incredibly talented producer of "GET FIT" at Prime Sports, Kurt Deichert, and my producer at Fox 4 News, Susan Grey.

My literary agent, Jan Miller, and her staff, in particular Ashley Carroll and Elizabeth Grant. They are the greatest in the world. Jan recognized a spark in me when I was a teenager. I was either too young or too dumb to recognize it in myself. Jan, thanks for believing.

I'd like to consider myself a good salesman and thank God for that, because it took a lot of selling to convince Skip Hollandsworth to ghost-write this book. Skip, you are simply the best, and thanks to your lovely wife, Shannon, for her support and help. To Gail Halperin and Colleen Glenn for their help in the stretching chapter. I want to thank Sally Stephenson for helping to write the cooking chapter. Lord knows that Skip and I would have burned it in the oven.

A special thanks to Simon & Schuster.

There are so many and you all know who you are, from my radio listeners to my gym members. I love you all and thank you for contributing to a book that I hope will help many people.

In April of 1989, I sat down behind a console at a Dallas radio station for my very first fitness call-in show. At the time, I was just another young trainer who had developed a reputation around the city for getting people into great shape. I thought my radio gig would be a great way to pass an afternoon—swapping information with other fitness types about weight-lifting, aerobic exercise, and low-fat food. It was going to be a hoot, an ego boost, a chance for me to show off everything I knew about the StairMaster and tricep pull-downs and abdominal crunches.

Five minutes into the show, I got my first phone call. "Larry," said a hesitant female voice: "All my life I've been called a success. And I've been one. I'm in my early 40s, I'm in a high-paying profession, I'm a good mother, a good wife—"

Then her voice faltered. "But no matter what I've done, there is one thing I live with every day. I feel sick walking out the door of my house because of my body. I've tried everything. I've done diets, I've taken diet pills, I've gone two hours straight on a treadmill. And I'm still over a hundred and seventy pounds. What I want to know is what can you possibly tell me that I haven't heard before?"

At that very moment, I was ready to throw away my how-to-do-the-perfect-bench-press. I wanted to spend the rest of my two-hour show talking to this woman, telling her that I knew exactly what she was going through. I wanted to tell her that I knew what it was like to starve myself until I wanted to weep, to do aerobics for hours until my knees were swollen to the size of softballs, to stare at myself in the mirror and wonder, "Why? Why does nothing change?" I wanted to tell her about the struggle that my own family had gone through, how my mother was one of the country's first members of Overeaters Anonymous, and how I had been a compulsive overeater myself.

But I also wanted to tell her that there was a *real* eating and exercise program that worked for *real* people, if only she would trust me to explain it to her. But here it was, my first day on the radio, with the producer in the control room waving frantically and the console lighting up manically. "Just stay with me," I told the woman. "If you listen to me for the next couple of hours, you'll understand exactly what it takes."

Praying that she would stay tuned, I went to the next caller— and found myself listening to another woman who said she was eating only one meal a day and still couldn't get rid of ten excess pounds. Then came a woman who told me she was staying thin, but couldn't give her body any shape. I stared at the console. There were more lights, more calls. "My God," I thought, "it's an epidemic." There was a man who told me he was a former high school sports star who got married after college, had a baby, and no longer knew how to motivate himself to work out again. Right behind him came a forty-year-old lawyer who told me he had put on fifty pounds over the last ten years, most of it around his mid-section. He told me he had tried five different diets in the last year. Quietly, I asked him how he felt. "Hopeless," he said. "My God, it's hopeless."

On my first day on radio, I was inundated by pleas for help. And since then, the pleas have never stopped. By now, I have taken tens of thousands of calls on my radio shows. I have received thousands more letters from my national television fitness show. I have consulted with or trained thousands who come to one of my health clubs. I have given more speeches and seminars than a traveling evangelist. Believe me, I have heard everything—every single myth and excuse that has kept you from getting the body you want, from women who have children and full-time jobs and who tell me they don't know when they can ever find the time to change their fitness habits to men who believe that if they lift weights two extra hours a week, they can eat whatever they want; women who are scared to lift any weights because they think it will make their muscles too big, and people who wonder why, if they're eating so much food that's labeled *nonfat*, they are still getting fatter.

What is astonishingly clear is that all of you are still confused about what it means to lose fat and get lean. Here we are, nearly at the dawn of the twenty-first century, and we are body-conscious to a degree unprecedented in human history. There are gleaming new gyms in every neighborhood. There are hordes of diet and fitness gurus. You can't flip through the television channels at night without coming across another fitness-fad infomercial telling you to buy another piece of "revolutionary" exercise equipment. And you can't open up a magazine without reading about a new kind of diet that another so-called expert swears will strip you of your excess weight.

Yet while surveys show that approximately half of the women and a quarter of the men in this country say they are on some sort of diet, government reports declare that Americans are gaining an average of one to two pounds a year. The average weight of an American woman under the age of thirty is seven pounds heavier than the weight of her counterpart in 1959. If you think about it, it's simply not true that we're turning into a nation of hard bodies. The reality is, according to the American Seating Company, that American fannies have widened by more than two inches in the last thirty years!

How could this have happened? Is it because we're just lazy and gluttonous? Of course not. All you have to do is listen to the pain in the voices of people who call me—people determined to succeed, yet utterly baffled that nothing is working. It breaks my heart to know how many of you try. I know about those of you who eat less—less!—than all of your co-workers at lunch, yet still have weight problems. I know how great your willpower has been, how courageous and dedicated you've been to dieting. And even as many times as these "medically supervised" diets have failed you, you can't help but be tempted by the next one that comes along. There's one that says if you eat a vat of cabbage soup, you'll lose seventeen pounds in a week. There's another telling you to eat more *fat* to lose weight. In the back of your mind, you're saying that none of this can be healthy for you. But you try it anyway. And you find that you may get artificially thin for a while. You begin to celebrate, then *boom!* The minute you get a wild craving for real food and start eating, you end up even fatter than before.

Then there's exercise. A few years ago, you were being told to participate in a high-impact aerobics class. Then you were told that your best body would only emerge if you took step, funk, power yoga, spinning, or kick-boxing classes—all of which seem enormously complicated. In the end, despite your best intentions, you feel like a greater failure because your body shape hasn't changed a bit.

WHO HAS REALLY FAILED?

Now listen to me. Before you read another word of this book, you have to get rid of the guilt that you have built up over the years about gaining weight or looking unshapely. What you must believe—and I mean *believe*—is that you have not failed in your old fitness and diet programs. Those programs have failed *you!* You have been duped. You have been misled most of your life with half-truths and outright lies about what fitness means.

Let me give you just a couple of examples. Instead of being honestly told what it takes to sculpt your body, you have been told that you must work out like an intense professional athlete. Instead of being taught what a true eating program is like, you have been told that weight loss will come only when you try to starve your body and thus shut down your body's engine. You think it's impossible to lose weight unless you go on a diet.

Diets! As you'll read in the next chapter, you are destined for

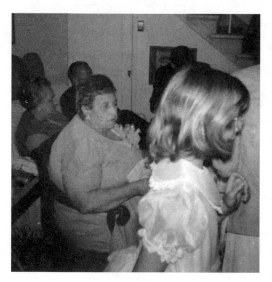

My grandmother, who was at one time close to 400 pounds.

failure every time you try to slow your body's engine. You are going to look worse if you remain fixated on losing weight instead of losing fat—a huge distinction. If you follow any diet, you may lose weight, but only temporarily. In the long run, you will become unhealthy, and your body will start malfunctioning.

Now, you may be thinking, why should I believe this, especially since plenty of doctors and nutritionists have written books based on one diet or another? Just remember, two things make me different from the other weight-loss gurus. First, like you, I've spent my life trying to find a program that worked. Before I created my own program, I was convinced I was genetically cursed to pile on the fat. I agonized over my body's tendency to put on weight. I did everything you have done, and more! I was like a lab rat. I took masses of diet pills. I went on laxative diets. I fasted, depriving my body of food for days at a time in order to look good for the beach; but once I got to the beach I found myself so ravenous that I couldn't stop eating. More than once I spent an entire day being "good," eating all the right foods, only to stand in front of the refrigerator late at night gorging my brains out. At one point, I decided to spend every waking moment at a gym, hoping I could look like Arnold Schwarzenegger, my childhood hero. Well, I got some big muscles, all right. But because I didn't know how to get the fat off my body, I was still too embarrassed to take my shirt off in public.

Then I began doing research. I studied the programs of the top fitness leaders in the country, and I began to put them to use to improve myself, as well as to train other people. The more I trained others, the more I realized what worked and what didn't. And that's the second reason I'm different from many diet-book authors. I developed a program the hard way, learning firsthand which fitness theories were exaggerated and which ones were myths. I don't pass along the advice of so-called experts unless I'm certain it works for people in the real world—people who aren't fitness fanatics but just want to feel good about their bodies.

For me, searching for the right program was like searching for the Holy Grail. Having grown up in a family of individuals who never felt good about their bodies, I became committed to giving people the right information. I knew that there were few worse feelings in the world than that feeling of self-consciousness about one's appearance.

Eventually, the program I put together began to have an impact. Hundreds of people came back to tell me that the program worked for them. After listening to my first day on the radio, the program director for that Dallas radio station started training with me and lost thirty-five pounds in eight weeks. Others knocked off ten, fifteen, twenty pounds in less time. And remember the first woman caller who weighed more than 170 pounds? I begged her to come to my gym and follow my eating program. She lost fifty pounds in four months.

Of course, every weight-loss program offers testimonials. What you want to know is that this program will work for you. So just remember one thing. All the people who have tried my program—even the ones who didn't lose much weight—later have told me that they could not believe how easy it was to change the shape and tone of their bodies. Why? Because my program is a way of life. It offers a simple, exact way to get a tighter stomach, sleeker hips, and firmly toned muscles in the legs and arms. When I worked out three times as hard as I now do, I didn't even come close to obtaining as well developed a body as I have since following what I now call the Larry North Program.

THE JOY OF CHANGE

I want you, too, to know that joy. With the North Program, you will learn to strip off fat and rediscover your sexier curves and muscles. Trust me, getting lean is going to make you feel far more exhilarated and successful than anything you've ever tried before. And unlike your experiences with most other programs, you'll never feel a need to quit. Even if you follow this program only halfway, you're going to see quick results. You're going to say, "Thank God, I've finally got it."

All I ask is that you be patient. My program—like anything that's worthwhile—is going to take a little time and concentration. It's going to take some motivation. But I will help you find that part of yourself that demands excellence. All you have to do for now is relax, and keep reading.

On the Larry North Program, you will see remarkable changes in yourself, and all without crazy, illogical diets and absurdly difficult workouts. My program—offering a very natural way to change your body—is one you can follow for the rest of your life. I've said this a thousand times, and I'll say it a thousand times more: Any program that you can't do for the rest of your life is not worth doing for a single day.

So congratulations. The past is behind you. You're about to have the most fun you've had in a very long time. As you'll discover, the North Program isn't a sacrifice, but a blessing.

Chapter One

THE MYTH OF DIETING: WHY DIETING MAKES YOU FATTER

I probably shouldn't say this, but I will be the first to admit that if you want to lose ten to twenty pounds quickly, just put this book down right now and start starving yourself. I promise you, with some effort you'll lose weight right away.

But study after study of dieters shows that almost all of you will not last two weeks on a diet. Most don't last a week. And here's the saddest news of all. If you do lose weight through diet

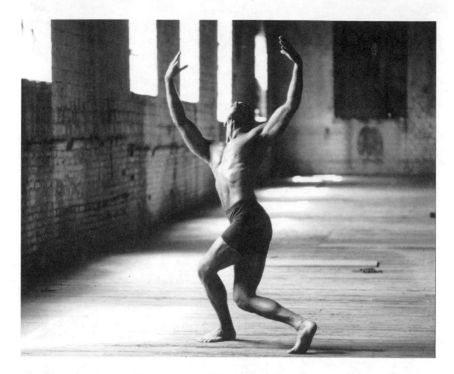

programs, you will gain it all back within a year. Here are the facts: There is simply no scientific evidence to suggest that dieting does anything other than create a temporary weight loss. Think about it. If losing weight were simply a matter of going on a diet—that is, cutting calories—then why aren't all of us able to do it? If all these diets really worked, then why are we collectively getting fatter?

Now I am not going to load you down with highly technical jargon about nutrition. But over the years, I have learned the one irrefutable science lesson that should make you forever abandon the idea of losing weight by starving yourself. What happens when you diet is that you force your body to slow down its *metabolism*, one of the most important words you're going to come across in this book.

Your metabolism is what burns calories to create energy. Think of it as your inner engine. The higher the level at which you can keep your engine revved up, the more fuel (or calories) it will burn. But if there is no fuel for your engine, your metabolism slows down. It tries to preserve every calorie it can. According to some studies, if you drop from 2,000 calories a day to 1,200, your metabolism decreases by 5 to 10 percent. If you drop to 800 calories a day, your metabolism lowers by a whopping 10 to 20 percent.

After a couple of weeks of a very strict diet, your body readjusts and starts cutting back on its own caloric needs. Suddenly, that paltry 800-calorie-a-day diet can feel like 8,000 calories. Because your metabolism is working at a snail's pace, you actually stop losing weight.

But that's not your only problem. With your slower metabolism rate, you're very vulnerable to gaining back huge amounts of weight. And you *will* gain it back, because at some point you will have to start eating again. You may think you're different, that you have the willpower to stop eating, but scientific research shows that when your body is starving, it is stronger than your brain. Your body will send such strong signals to your brain that you will break into Fort Knox if there's a candy bar in there. Come on, you know it's true. If you diet, you will also overeat.

And the minute you start eating again, two things will happen to you. First, your depleted carbohydrate cells, desperate to soak up any fluid they can, will act like sponges and regain every bit of water weight that you lost during your diet; and second, your slowed metabolic rate won't be able to speed up in time to burn off the new food you have just put in, which means the food will go right to your fat cells.

"Hold on," you say, "I thought I had gotten rid of my fat cells when I dieted!"

Sorry, you've been duped again. For the most part, what you lose when you diet is your muscle tissue—the most valuable part of your body for maintaining a high metabolic rate. Granted, your body will pull calories from some of your fat cells, but it will first look to your muscles for nourishment. The truth is that your body *wants* to get rid of your muscle tissue. Why? In its diet-starvation mode, your body, desperate to preserve itself, is doing everything it can to save calories, not burn them. And what's the one thing that burns calories? Your muscles! Fat is metabolically inactive because its function is to serve as a big old greasy warehouse for the storage of fat cells. In other words, fat tissue does nothing but collect fat. Muscle tissue, on the other hand, is the critical element in maintaining a high metabolism. It's what makes your body act like a powerful furnace, burning up the calories that come in. It follows, then, that the fewer muscles in your body, the less food fuel you need to consume. Some studies say that up to 50 percent of the weight you lose on a diet will come from your muscles, the very component of your body you should keep and build to keep the weight off. On top of that, when you diet, your body can potentially double the number of its fat storage enzymes to hoard more calories. Visualize *that*—multiplying fat cells!—while you're starving yourself.

At the end of a diet, you end up with shrunken muscle cells and a higher percentage of body fat. You're fatter! Instead of weighing 160 pounds with 30 percent body fat, for example, your diet has dropped you to 135 pounds but given you 40 percent body fat.

Wait. The nightmare continues. When your diet fails and you start eating again, your body fat is going to get even higher, because all that food is going straight to your fat cells. Without an exercise plan, you're not developing muscle to burn it up. So now you have even more fat to lose in your next diet! And the cycle begins again.

You've probably noticed that every time you go on another diet, it takes longer for your body to lose the weight and it regains weight faster. In frustration, you might turn to one of these "new, improved" lines of diet pills, hoping to jump-start your weight loss. Sure enough, your weight goes down—for a while. But if you don't know how to eat or exercise correctly, you won't know how to achieve permanent results.

More bad news. If you have certain problem areas, dieting only make them more problematic. Fat, it has been said, is like a river. It flows right to that part of the body that offers the least resistance. In men, it goes to the middle, creating those dreaded pot bellies. In women, it goes to the buttocks and thighs. In other words, dieting does not reshape your problem areas. It makes them worse.

THE PSYCHOLOGICAL HELL OF DIETING

What else do you need to know? I've seen people who have been on so many low-calorie diets that they have a medically dangerous fat-to-muscle ratio. Furthermore, such a yoyo pattern of dieting—losing and regaining, losing and regaining—significantly increases the risk of heart disease. And even if you don't die of a heart attack, you'll be so sick from your starvation that you won't be able to enjoy life.

And that's what bothers me most. Ultimately, a diet does nothing but make you deeply unhappy. You can't enjoy the life around you, because you're obsessing about not eating. Yet the more you obsess, the more you think and dream about food.

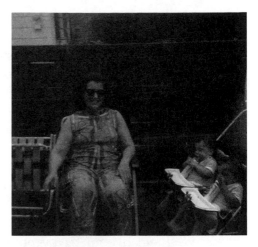

My mom at the time in her life when she hated her body.

I know firsthand just what a disturbing emotional issue dieting can be. My mother spent most of her life consumed with worry over her weight. By the time she was six years old, my mother was the fattest kid in her neighborhood. When she was eleven, her mother, who then weighed nearly 300 pounds, took her to her first diet doctor. The doctor prescribed diet pills and two boxes of appetite suppressant chocolate candy. By the time she got home, my mother had eaten all the candy in both boxes. Although she was considered a jolly, cheerful girl, she cried herself to sleep.

It didn't get any better when she reached adulthood. By then, she was so addicted to diet pills that she needed them just to stay awake through the day. She would take her pills all week and try not to eat, then binge all through the weekend. She was in the very first Overeaters Anonymous chapter in the country. She joined Weight Watchers. She sent off for every weight-loss program advertised in the backs of magazines. She tried a diet that required daily injections. After trying the Beverly Hills Diet, she went around for days with her lips puckered from the pineapples recommended in the program. She tried diuretics and laxatives. She wore rubber gloves when preparing food, because she had been told that fat from meat could get into her pores and prevent her from losing weight.

As a young boy, I felt that I was in a madhouse. One afternoon, I was out with my mother and bought a hot dog with my carefully earned money. My mother was on one of her typical

500-calories-a-day diets. I hadn't even take a bite of that hot dog when she shouted, "Larry, look over there! There's your father!" As I turned around, my mother grabbed the hot dog and stuck the whole thing in her mouth. The whole thing! I started crying, and so did my mom. She was crying over what this absurd life of dieting had done to her—a life that would drive her to steal her own child's treat.

When people ask me why I'm in this business, I tell this story. My mother never knew what it was like to sit by the side of a swimming pool and feel comfortable. She thought no man would ever want her because of her ugly legs. Her weight had a stranglehold on her whole life.

I feel a pain in my heart whenever I tell the story of my mother. Yet because of her, I am devoted to making sure no one else has to go through that same torture.

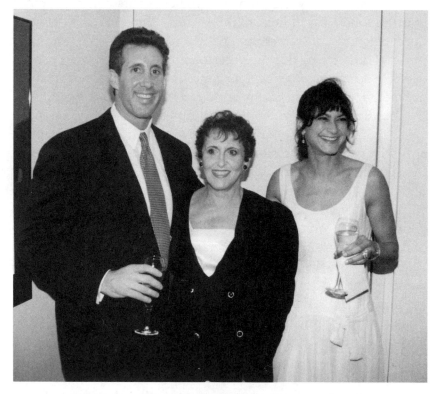

Mom, with me and my wife Melanie twenty years later—
and more than forty pounds lighter.

BREAKING FREE FROM THE FAT COCOON

But there is an answer. A few years ago, my younger brother Alan was telling me in our long-distance conversations that he was in great shape, so I invited him to move to Dallas to help run my new gym. But when Alan stepped off the plane, I was speechless. What could I say? He was a North, prone to get heavy at the drop of a hat. He had tried everything the rest of us had tried—and yet he kept getting heavier and heavier. Although he'd been too ashamed to tell me, he weighed more than 300 pounds, 120 pounds more than his twin brother.

At that moment I told myself, if I can't help my own brother, I don't have a right to help anyone else. I took him to lunch and said, "Get ready." I ordered him a chicken breast grilled with no oil, a cup of rice, and a side dish of vegetables. He said, "Larry, how am I going to lose weight eating all this food?" I replied, "Alan, this is the program. You're going to be eating these kinds of meals all the time. You're going to lift weights and do some cardio work. You're going to learn to feed your muscles and starve your fat."

He looked at me. "What?" he said. "I'm going to what?"

"Feed the muscles and starve the fat."

Four months later, Alan had dropped 100 pounds and had become one of the most popular and knowledgeable trainers in the gym, now rated one of the best in the country by *Vogue* magazine. He changed because he trusted me, even though at first the program didn't make sense to him. If you ever want to get and stay permanently lean, I told him, you have to start focusing on your muscle tissue. I'm not talking here about bulky pumping-iron muscle. I'm talking about the skeletal muscle within your body. It's your fountain of youth, your gold at Fort Knox. It is what stokes your body's metabolism so that you can burn off the food you eat and shrink your fat reserves. Nothing is going to rejuvenate that metabolism except lean, silky, beautiful muscle—not dieting, not liposuction, not diet pills, not an extra hour a day on a treadmill, not even a five-day-a-week running program.

As I'll explain later, if you focus on nothing but aerobics and cardiovascular exercise, you will not permanently speed up your metabolism. Sure, you'll burn calories—sometimes in the form of fat and sometimes in the form of carbohydrates. But the fact is that your body burns most of its fat during the day when you're *not* working out. It burns more total calories when you're walking around, doing your work, even when you're just sitting around and breathing. So it follows that if your body is full of highly toned muscle tissue, you'll burn far more calories throughout the day, because your metabolic rate is so much higher.

And that, in essence, is the key to the North Program. In my program, you must eat the kinds of food that build muscle tissue and keep your metabolism working. The other component of the eating program is meal frequency, which makes your metabolism work even faster. Finally, you'll want to build your muscles naturally through careful weight training (not a fanatical regimen of weight lifting). Think of it as body shaping, not body building.

And here's the best part of this story. You'll see results quickly, because you will feel your muscles starting to work inside you. Building muscle tissue doesn't take years. It begins the day you start the program.

Still skeptical? Afraid I might send you to the gym to grunt and groan for hours under a bench press? Wrong again. We're going to start with food, because proper eating makes up 70 to 80 percent of the North Program.

So let's get started. It's time to reveal the thin from within!

C h a p t e r   T w o

REAL FOOD:
EATING YOUR WAY TO
A BEAUTIFUL BODY

Here's what happens when you eat food: Some of it enters your bloodstream and is used as an energy source. The rest is stored either in your muscle cells or your fat cells. When your fat cells store food, that food turns into fat. But the food that gets into your muscle cells operates as fuel. Clearly, your goal is to get food to by-pass your fat cells and head to your muscles. But how do you do that? First you need to understand the difference between

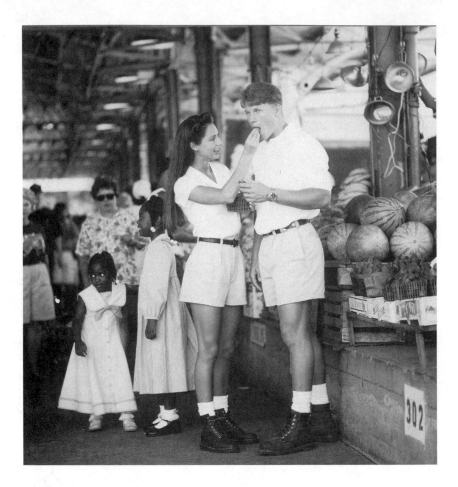

fuel for muscles and food for fat: Your muscle tissue takes in certain amounts of only the highest quality food nutrients. While fat cells will accept anything, your muscle tissue is very particular. It requires the best proteins and complex carbohydrates that you can find. What's more, it requires those proteins and carbs throughout the day in certain regulated amounts.

More people are confused by this concept than just about anything else I know when it comes to eating. They believe that if they eat low-fat or nonfat food, the food won't turn into fat, and that one massive dinner of very nutritious food fuels their muscles for the day.

Wrong! The cells in your muscles can only handle a certain amount of food at a time. After that, the cells shut their doors and don't allow any more food in, no matter how nutritious it is, until they have burned up or digested the food already there. So where does that excess food go? You guessed it. Straight to your fat cells.

That's why eating a large meal a day simply doesn't work. You may think you can eat a huge lunch and then skip dinner, so your body can work through all the extra food you ate. But that's not the way your body works. A big meal swamps the digestive system. If you eat 1,000 calories in one sitting, your body might only be able to handle 600 of them. The remaining amount will be stored as fat.

MEAL FREQUENCY

Now let's think back for a minute. In the previous chapter, I told you it's bad not to eat. And here I am in this chapter telling you it's bad *to* eat, even if it's "good food." Is there any hope? Of course there is. Just like my brother Alan, you're going to learn to feed the muscle and starve the fat.

Remember what I told you about thinking of your body as a finely tuned engine. Just like your car engine, it needs regular fill-ups of fuel, and the fuel must be of the highest octane. That's why the North Program recommends eating five meals a day (maybe six if you're male). Each meal is completely balanced, composed of a protein and a carbohydrate, with a fibrous vegetable added when it's convenient. I know when I present it this way, it sounds impossible—totally undoable. But be patient. As you'll see in Chapter Five, I'm going to show you a myriad of ways to prepare your foods so that you don't think you're eating the same old thing every time. But the first thing you need to understand about the North Program is that meal frequency is a cornerstone to the plan for success. It's important to eat a meal of those foods your muscles crave.

I know this idea—getting lean by eating more meals each day—turns traditional diet thinking on its head. But the theory that our days should consist of three meals—breakfast, lunch, and dinner—is wildly outdated. If you eat only three meals per day, you're keeping food from your body for up to six hours at a time. Your body will be so famished that by the time you take in food again that you will overeat. As I'm sure you know, undereating always leads to overeating. Skipping or missing meals will set off an increased craving in your body for the very foods that you're trying to avoid.

Let's say you're trying to get lean, and you have a cup of coffee and toast for breakfast. Then you eat a salad and yogurt for lunch. Then you go from 1:00 P.M. to 7:00 P.M. without eating. When you walk into the house, exhausted and hungry, what do you think you're going to want to eat? Certainly not a grilled chicken breast with steamed broccoli and brown rice. You're going to want fatty foods and sugar—the very things your muscles will never take in. This craving is a physical need, not just a psychological one. Your body is shutting down and requires energy— and sugar is one of the quickest ways to get it. The reason you crave something fatty is that you want food that is instantly satisfying, that fills you up quickly.

That's why frequent meals, all of them spaced throughout the day, are critically important. If you consume four to six meals a day (four or five for women, six for men), you'll have more energy because your blood sugar level remains stable. And because you're eating regularly, you'll never feel that you're starving or that you'll lose control when you sit down for a meal. Breaking up meals also allows your body to work best at absorbing the necessary nutrients. Your metabolism can better handle protein, for example, if the protein is broken into smaller amounts throughout the day. At the beginning, it may seem that you are eating even when you're not hungry (another dieters' taboo). But once you're up to speed on the program, your body will metabolize the meals so efficiently that you will be hungrier more often. Don't worry, it's a great sign!

If you follow this meal plan, you speed up your all-important metabolism. You're sending into your engine pure injections of fuel at regular intervals. Just as putting too much wood on a fire can snuff it out, putting too much food into your body can slow down the engine. Feeding the fire regularly is the key. When you eat a huge meal, you become more sedentary. After such a meal, a great amount of blood is drawn to the digestive tract to try to absorb the food. That means less blood goes to the brain and the muscles, which means you have less energy. You turn into one of those post-feasting zombies.

THE NORTH PROGRAM FOODS

If you're really a skeptic, you're thinking, "Larry North might be talking a good game about meal frequency, but what he's really going to make me do is eat tiny, tiny meals at inconvenient times."

But actually, when you first begin on the North Program, you will not be able to imagine that you can eat this much food. You'll wonder, "How can I eat so much protein and carbohydrates in one day?" Well, as I mentioned, if you follow the North Program closely, hunger is the sign of success. It means the food you're sending to your muscle tissue is getting burned up by your metabolism, so you're going to be ready for your next meal sooner than you think. Isn't that idea alone enough to make you want to change all your attitudes toward eating? Instead of pretending to have no appetite, instead of trying to ignore your hunger signals, you can eat abundantly, because that's what healthy people are supposed to do. You'll know you are a success at this program when you are always hungry, always eating the right meals, and you still can't keep any weight on your body. (Believe me, it will happen!)

Furthermore, with the North Program, you don't have to waste your time counting calories and fat grams (as if there is any way for you to figure out how many calories are in every single morsel of food you eat). The North Program makes your life much easier by showing you how to pick the right amounts of foods from three food groups. At each meal, you want a starchy complex carbohydrate (also known as a *carb*), which provides the basic energy for your body. Carbs are the most efficiently burned foods you can take in. A protein is also critical at each meal, because it provides the amino acids necessary to keep muscle. Protein becomes even more important as you begin the weight training portion of the program, because you need to replenish the muscles you exercise. Finally, fibrous vegetables are necessary in your diet (although not at every meal), not only because they are full of vitamins, but because they also help the digestive system operate smoothly. And because they are digested more slowly, they help you to feel full more quickly.

Of course, your body does require some fat, in the form of the "essential fatty acids." Fat serves as an insulator for your body and also as a lubricator for your joints. But you do not need to eat fatty foods to get those essential fatty acids. Since the food groups I've already mentioned contain enough natural fat in them to provide what you need, you don't need to add any more fat to your diet. In truth, with every extra pound of fat you take in, you're adding extra blood vessels to your body—miles of them. These blood vessels draw away the very blood you need to move through your other body organs.

NORTH PROGRAM FOOD SELECTIONS

You can choose from among any of these foods:

Complex Carbohydrates: These include brown rice, yams, grits, white potatoes, sweet potatoes, oatmeal, oat bran, corn, whole-grain breads, whole-grain pastas, shredded wheat, cream of rice, beans, black-eyed peas, lima beans, black beans, white beans, pinto beans, and many more.

Proteins: These include cuts of boneless, skinless turkey breast, white meat of chicken, white fish, egg whites, lean venison and other game meats, the very leanest cuts of beef like sirloin, eye of round steak, pork center tenderloin, and canned tuna, chicken, or turkey in water. (Make sure to look at the labels of canned tuna. Because tuna is migratory fish, it will contain more fat when caught at certain times of year. Don't buy a can of tuna that's got six grams of fat per serving. Look for cans with only one gram of fat.)

Fibrous vegetables: These include broccoli, cauliflower, carrots, green and red peppers, asparagus, celery, spinach, lettuces, green peas, tomatoes, eggplant, green beans, squash, cabbage, radishes, onions, zucchini, cucumbers, and many more.

Fruits: If you are intent on getting as lean as you can, you will want to reduce your fruit intake, because it contains sugar. However, eating a piece as a snack or as part of one of your daily meals isn't going to hurt your program. The best fruits (meaning lower in sugar) are strawberries, apples, pears, and berries. In second place, but still okay, are grape-fruits, cantaloupe, mangoes, tangerines, oranges, honey-dew, papayas, plums, and nectarines. Fruits like bananas, pineapples, peaches, grapes and watermelon are very high in sugar, so they should be avoided.

So your eating program needs to consist of one serving of a carb (with no butter or fatty sauces), one of a protein (grilled, broiled, or baked, with no oil), and an occasional fibrous veg-etable. That's it. If you follow this program, the weight will melt off you so fast your head will spin.

WHAT DO I AVOID?

Don't be one of these people who gets caught up in the theory that you've got to cut down the amount of all foods to lose weight. Not all calories are created equal, and the fewer calories you have coming from fatty food, the better off you are.

Just this once, I'm going to do some calorie counting for you to prove a point. When you ingest one gram of fat, you're taking in nine calories. That's more than twice as many calories as come from a gram of a carbohydrate or a gram of protein. In other words, you can afford to eat more if you're eating the right foods. If you eat, say, only 1,000 calories a day, but they're coming from high-fat foods like potato chips and ice cream, then those "fat calories" (calories that come from fatty food) will go straight to your fat cells. Some studies even say that 97 percent of all fat calo-ries you take in will be converted into body fat.

So what exactly do I mean by fatty foods?

Oils: Try to keep oil to a bare minimum. That includes salad dressings, vegetable cooking oils, cooking sprays, butter, mayonnaise, sour cream, and margarine. It's oil that makes fried food so fattening, which is why you should stay away from anything fried. A single tablespoon of that oil contains 120 calories of fat—a tablespoon! Look for monosaturated and polyunsaturated oils, but remember, the less oil the better.

Sugar: Obviously, you want to get rid of simple sugars, like the sugar in candies and soft drinks, because they can go straight into your bloodstream (and your fat cells). That's why they are called "empty calories." You know which products have sugar. Try to cutdown on all forms of sugar in your food intake. Four grams equal one teaspoon, and one twelve-ounce soft drink has forty grams, so you're getting ten tea-spoons of sugar in each soda!

Dairy: You want to make your dairy products a treat, not a staple. It's virtually impossible to lose fat while consuming any array of cheeses or milk. Whole milk contains 49.2 percent fat calories. Two percent milk means you're getting two percent less fat than in whole milk. That's *all* it means. You're still getting more than 40 percent fat. Nonfat milk is acceptable, but don't overdo it.

Processed foods: This means about anything that comes in a box or package, such as cold cuts, crackers, chips, packaged macaroni, frozen waffles, pancake mixes, peanut butter, pastas, white flour products, cereal, and bread. Some processed foods are good sources of starchy carbs, but by the time they are mixed, mashed, and boxed, they become calorically dense. Your body can't handle them all. Almost all processed foods have loads of added oil, sodium, or sugar. I don't want you to think that breads and pastas and cereals are bad for you. They're just extremely high in calories. One serving size of pasta, just two ounces, is 210 calories, which is about 50 more calories than a medium-sized baked potato. But very few people sit down to two ounces of pasta. They typically eat six to eight ounces at one meal. That's when pasta becomes a poor choice. Likewise, if you want to get lean, bread is one of the first things you need to reduce. A bagel is so packed with condensed flour that just one of them can contain more than 400 calories! One plain bagel (without any jelly or butter or, God forbid, cream cheese) has as many calories as ten egg whites and a cup of oatmeal.

Fatty Meats: Again, this should be a no-brainer. We're talking about bacon, sausage, hot dogs (over 50 percent of a hot dog's calories comes from fat!), corn dogs, beef jerky, fish sticks, and sardines. Also, be careful of dark meat chicken and turkey. Dark meat chicken is over 40 percent fat, while white meat chicken is only 4 to 10 percent fat. And be careful of darker meat fish like salmon, which is 44 percent fat. Also be wary of deli meats. They are not as healthy a protein source, because they've been processed. And some of them, when processed, get loaded with extra fat. Remember, your muscles want high-quality, low-fat food.

High-fat natural foods: Just because a food is classified as natural doesn't mean you get lean by eating it. Such foods as avocados, coconuts, olives, nuts, and seeds are mostly 80 percent fat. Avoid dried fruits like raisins (which have 210 calories per half cup.) Also stay away from certain "health foods" that can be the most fat-laden substances around. Six ounces of tofu contain a whopping sixteen grams of fat. Natural peanut butter has more fat than regular peanut butter. And granola is ridiculously high in fat. Just because a food is healthy does not mean it gets you lean.

AM I LEFT WITH ANYTHING TO EAT?

No doubt some of you are panicking, thinking, "Carbs, proteins, and fibrous vegetables are all I can eat for the rest of my life?" But if you look over my suggested food list again, you'll find that you're eating most of those foods already. In effect, very little is being removed from your usual choices of foods, except perhaps dessert. And as I am going to explain in a minute, the North Program does allow for some cheating. Although you'll get leaner if you follow the program strictly, you'll still see substantial results if you follow the eating program only 50 percent of the way, because you've finally made a healthy decision for your body.

But, you think, "How can I live without my favorite fat-laden foods? I need taste!" Well, you'll have to give that excuse up. I've been with people who would interrupt me before I even got the chance to explain the eating program, because they thought the food they'd have to eat was so "boring." They would tell me that my program is about boiled chicken, steamed rice, and no flavor.

Sorry, but they only imagined the food would be boring. On the North Program, you're eating the same foods as always. You're just going to prepare them slightly differently, which I'll explain in Chapter Five. Imagine this: You have one shot glass full of cooking oil, another glass full of melted butter, another full of salad dressing, and one full of sugar. All the North Program does is take those shot glasses out of your diet. Just by removing some fat, some sugar, and some processed foods, you make sure your body is receiving only foods that can be burned efficiently by your internal engine.

So you've got to stop thinking that healthy food is bland food. That's just a crummy excuse to eat more junk. Let me give you some great examples of substitutes for fatty foods:

Dairy: Skim milk, nonfat sour cream, nonfat yogurt, nonfat cheese, nonfat cottage cheese, egg beaters, and egg whites (all the fat of an egg is in the yolk: the white has pure protein and no fat).

Dressings and Sauces: There are so many different nonfat condiments these days to add flavor to your food that I have an entire refrigerator at my home filled with nothing but condiments. To name a few: Tabasco, picante sauce, yellow and Dijon mustard, seasoned vinegars, balsamic and wine vinegars, canned tomato paste, horseradish, canned fat-free sauces, fat-free dressings, and soy sauces.

Freezer Foods: There are also very nutritional frozen foods, from frozen berries to frozen vegetables to fat-free frozen hash browns (bake them instead of frying them, and you won't be able to tell the difference).

Juices: Look for lemon juice, lime juice, Crystal Light, and other flavored beverages that contain no sugar or fat.

Chips/snacks: How many low-fat potato chips are on the market these days? If you can't stand the new breed of low-fat chips and desperately need a salty snack, go with pretzels. There is also a great array of sugar-free and fat-free puddings and popsicles. If you want popcorn, make sure it's air-popped and not prepared with cooking oil. (Remember, "natural flavored popcorn" usually has no less fat than butter-flavored.)

I'm not going to play games with you. As much publicity and advertising as there may be about the fat-free foods hitting the market, let me warn you that those, too, contain mostly empty calories that will never get to your muscles. And because you read it's free of fat, you're more likely to eat a larger quantity of it.

I once had a wealthy business executive come into my gym, pay the initiation fee, and head off to work out. After three months, he stormed into my office and demanded his money back.

"I've followed your entire program," he said, "and I've gained fifteen pounds and added three inches to my waist. This isn't what I was promised!"

"Time out," I said. "Tell me what you're eating." My client described a very good eating program. He told me he was working out three to five times a week, thirty to sixty minutes each time. I was perplexed. "Is there any kind of snack you might be having?" I asked.

"Well, yeah, I eat fat-free cookies, but I know that doesn't count."

"How many?"

"Just a couple of boxes a day."

I nearly leaped out of my seat. "Bob," I sputtered, "with those cookies, you're taking in eighteen hundred calories of garbage a day. Because you're following my eating program, you're giving the muscle everything it wants. So those cookies are going straight to your fat cells. Those two boxes are the equivalent of five meals a day. Fat-free doesn't mean calorie-free. It doesn't keep fat off your body!"

Bob had forgotten the lesson of my program: You must feed the muscle and starve the fat. Once he stopped sabotaging his program with fat-free junk, he shaped up and lost weight.

Yet even now, as convinced as you might be by what I've said so far, I know what your dark little mind is thinking. "Larry," you're asking, "how exactly do you expect me to eat so many balanced meals a day?"

It's time to turn the page.

Chapter Three

FREE OF FAT FOR LIFE: EATING THE LARRY NORTH WAY

People who get started on my program never think they can squeeze in so many meals a day considering how busy they are and how many responsibilities they have. I've heard all these excuses a thousand times, and I always say, "Let me take out my violin." The truth of the matter is that most of you are already eating five times a day. What you're ignoring is the caloric impact of the little sixty-second "snacks" that you have in the midmornings and midafternoons. You're also forgetting about that quick graze in front of the refrigerator right before you go to bed at night.

Let's just go through the day of a typical person and see how much he really eats.

Breakfast: Let's assume, just to be on the safe side, that our average guy skips breakfast altogether, because he's trying to lose weight or he's in a hurry for work. No way he'll get in five meals on this day, right? Guess again.

Midmorning: Coffee and a bran muffin. He thinks a bran muffin is healthy, because it's got bran in it. It probably also contains 400 calories, with ten to fifteen grams of fat.

Lunch: A standard lunch at a restaurant near work, anything from a club sandwich to Mexican food. If he's trying to be good, he'll eat a turkey sandwich.

Midafternoon: A candy bar, pack of potato chips, or piece of fruit. If it's been a bad day, he'll have all three.

After work: Doesn't every person in America have a quick snack, perhaps chips and hot sauce, before dinner?

Dinner: A traditional meal of a meat, potatoes, vegetables, salad, a dessert, and wine. Huge caloric overload.

Late-night snack: David Letterman has some great guests on, so our guy stays up with ice cream or a bowl of cereal. Because he feels guilty about eating so late, he decides to skip breakfast the next day, so his body will have time to work through all the food he's eaten the previous day.

That, my friends, is a six-meal day. If you eat like that 365 days a year, you're going to pile on the fat! But if you knock out some of the fat meals and snacks and add a better balance of proteins and carbs, your body will change in a hurry. And instead of allowing your emotional and physical stamina to plummet throughout the day, you'll feel terrific, because your body is well fueled.

Now let me take you through an average day for me:

Breakfast, 8:00 A.M.: A bowl of oatmeal, two pieces of dry toast (I add jelly), and an omelet made of egg whites and veggies (no added fat).

Midmorning, 11:00 A.M.: A turkey sandwich and steamed rice prepared at home and brought with me to work.

Lunch, 2:00 P.M.: Grilled chicken (or a grilled white meat turkey burger), a baked potato with salsa topping, and a salad with fat-free dressing.

Midafternoon, 5:00 P.M.: After a workout, six to eight hard-boiled eggs, a package of baby carrots, a bottle of purified water, and two slices of honeydew melon (a meal, incidentally, that costs less than five dollars).

Dinner, 8:30 P.M.: A cheeseless pizza with chicken, peppers, and mushrooms.

Late-night, 11:00 P.M.: A snack of fat-free chocolate pudding with a cup of yogurt and one scoop of a protein powder mixed in the yogurt.

In terms of time, some of these meals last no longer than ten minutes. (Incidentally, it doesn't lower the amount of calories in the food if you take the time to chew each bite 25 times versus 10 times.) But what's really important is that I am being sure to eat a proper balance of proteins and carbs at each of my meals. I see a lot of people hurting their program by overdosing at one meal on nothing but carbs, overwhelming their bodies with protein the next meal, then just eating a big salad at another meal. What's more, I see other people who eat nothing but pasta or other carbs and wonder why they aren't losing weight. I see yet others go the opposite way, eating as few carbs as possible, and still not losing weight.

Once again, all you have to do is visualize your body. If you eat a lot of carbs at a single meal, your muscle will take what carbs it needs, then send the rest on to your fat cells. It'll do the same thing if it's given too much protein at one time. On the other hand, if your carb intake is too low, your craving for sugar goes through the roof, and you'll develop an uncontrollable craving for a candy bar or other fat-laden food. Granted, some of you will temporarily lose some weight by reducing your carb intake. But what you're losing is largely water weight, which comes right back the moment you start eating carbs again.

Ultimately, what you want your body to do is maintain what nutritionists call a positive nitrogen balance. I don't want to get too technical; what you really need to know is that to sharpen your muscle tone, you must have a positive nitrogen balance. This is achieved through frequent protein feedings, with carbohydrates, throughout the day. Proteins with carbs help stabilize your blood sugar, keep you satisfied for longer periods of time, and increase your metabolic rate. Indeed, if you get your body accustomed to receiving similar amounts of food every three hours, your metabolism will become much more effective.

HOW MUCH FOOD SHOULD I EAT?

Now we come to our next thorny issue—knowing what amount of food constitutes an adequate meal for you.

To keep this as simple as possible, visualize a round dinner plate and divide the plate into three compartments for a protein, a carb, and a fibrous vegetable. if you're a man, you'll probably need larger quantities of food. A man tends to need five to eight ounces of a protein at each meal (an ounce is about two full bites of meat put into the average-sized mouth), while a woman needs three to five ounces (a portion that would look roughly like the size of a deck of playing cards). You want a cup to a cup and a half of carbs for each serving and one to three cups of a fibrous vegetable per serving. A cup of food, for those of you who don't have a measuring cup in your house, is about the amount of food you can put in a regular-sized coffee cup—and no fair squishing tons of food into a mug, now!

Depending on your body type, you may have to keep your portions smaller; you may discover that the quantities I recommend are more than you normally eat. Eat what you can. From now on you are eating your way to a beautiful body.

If you are one of those die-hards who must count calories, here is an efficient way to figure out what your intake should be. If you are a physically inactive person who doesn't work out, multiply your body weight by 12. If you weigh 200 pounds, for example, multiply 200 times 12 for a total of 2,400. Then divide that number by 5 (for five meals a day), and that should give you the average total number of calories you should be eating at each meal. Remember to include a protein and a carb at each meal.

If you're a moderately active person, multiply your body weight by 17, then divide by 5 to get your average number of calories per meal.

If you're very active—someone who runs marathons, works construction, or is on her feet all day taking care of three kids—you might very well multiply your body weight by 25 and then divide by 5 for your caloric intake per meal. Of course, these are just guidelines. Above all, you need to get to know your body. If you are a naturally muscular person who does minimal exercise and still has a great body, then you are a *mesomorph* and you don't have to be fanatically strict about the North Program. If you tend to be on the round side and put on weight easily, you're an *endomorph* and need to be especially dedicated to meal frequency and proper portions, so you don't end up bingeing. If you're naturally tall and skinny, with long limbs, you're an *ectomorph*. Your body is naturally geared to burn energy in overdrive and retain little weight. You can get away with eating more fat, but you'll also find the North Program beneficial, since it encourages you to eat more protein, the fuel for building muscles and giving your body the shape and contour you want.

Finally, here's how to determine if you need to increase or decrease calories:

A. You know you're working the program correctly when your waistline gets smaller and your energy level and strength continue to increase.

B. If your waistline is getting smaller but your energy level is decreasing proportionately, then you're probably undereating. This doesn't mean you should add fat. Simply add more carbs and protein to your meals.

C. If your waistline is growing and your energy level is still great, then clearly you are eating too much. You need to shave your portion sizes.

D. If you aren't sure how your body is responding, don't panic. Stay with the program and eat moderately but enough to be satisfied. Remember to make the distinction between "satisfied" and "full." If you're trying to gauge how much to eat, stop halfway through a meal, put down your silverware, and ask, "How hungry am I right now? How much more do I really need or want to eat?"

THE GREAT SECRET: PREPARING YOUR FOOD

One more thing before you begin your first day on the North Program. The key to the whole eating program is that you must have access to the right foods when it's time for you to eat. If you don't have these foods at your fingertips, you'll either start eating food that's terrible for you or missing meals.

The secret is that you must prepare your food ahead of time. If you don't have larger quantities of food prepared for at least some of your meals each day, you'll drive yourself crazy. Preparing meals before you need them saves you tremendous time and money, and anybody with minimal cooking experience can learn to bake, broil, and grill. If you follow my suggestions, you'll be able to leave your house each day, as I do, with little containers of the right foods, so you won't end up heading to the vending machine or some fast-food restaurant in the middle of the day.

Although I'm going to discuss how to prepare a stunning variety of healthy, tasty meals in Chapter Five, I want to give you a brief example of how I can make up a week's worth of the right kinds of food in a couple of hours:

I pop a dozen chicken breasts and/or fish fillets on the grill— and I'm done. I store the food I will eat the first three days in the refrigerator. I put the rest in the freezer and thaw it the night before I'm going to eat it. I reheat or microwave it, add vegetables, and I'm ready for a meal. Although I eat a couple of meals each day at restaurants (because I know how to order, which I will teach you to do in Chapter Five), I always carry along a plastic container of the food that I've prepared so I can squeeze in meals at work or on the road.

"But Larry," you say, "what you're suggesting is not what I'd call gourmet eating."

So what? Are you telling me that you eat a magnificent meal

every time you sit down at the table? For the North Program to work correctly, you have to eat frequent meals, and this is the best way to do it. Besides, since you're preparing your own food, you will know you're eating as healthfully as possible. You won't have to leap from your desk several times a day to search for the right food. You won't get cravings that keep you thinking about food all the time. And if you're the type who feels it's inconvenient or a little embarrassing to bring a container of food to your office, then you need to ask yourself what's most important to you. Is it preferable, for instance, to pull out your "fat clothes" on days when you feel heavy? Trust me, once you get into the habit of bringing your own food with you each day, it's no different from making sure you've got your keys.

BAD CHOICES AS PART OF A GOOD CHOICES PLAN

I'm going to present you with a six-week plan to learn to eat the Larry North way, which will start easily and eventually get tougher. I'm not going to demand a lifetime commitment. I'm just asking you to try it for a few weeks. Don't expect yourself to be 100 percent successful right away. After all, it takes a while to change bad eating habits. In fact, taking it slow is only going to help you. And remember this very important fact: If you miss a meal or overindulge at one meal, don't feel stricken and revert to poor eating habits. You haven't blown the program. All you have to do is pick right back up where you left off. By the sixth week, you'll know what it's like to get your body's metabolism fired up to its prime level.

As odd as it sounds, part of your journey to eating the Larry North way is knowing how to cheat, or treat. As you'll see, I encourage cheat meals. I am a realist, and I know no one—not even I—can follow this program all the time. Most people can only go so long depriving themselves of their very favorite fat foods. So if you include some of those foods as part of your program, you have the comfort of knowing that you won't fail in a massive way. Of course, this should not mean you can declare that you're going to have a cheat meal and gorge at a pizza buffet for hours. Even when you cheat, you need to exercise some portion control. Cheating is not an excuse to binge.

It's been my experience with clients that as they finally learn to eat correctly and develop the North Body, they don't want to return to their old greasy or fried foods. They actually lose the taste for their cheat foods. While you may not believe it now, I'm sure the same thing will happen to you. This program is not about being perfect. It's about making progress.

BETTER BAD CHOICES

A critical technique you should learn is how to make "better bad choices" a term I'm borrowing from Keith Klein. If you decide to cheat, there are foods you can pick that won't make you leaner but will prevent you from getting fatter. Let's say you're at a sporting event, concert, or movie theater—someplace where you're stuck with a very fixed menu, almost all of it high in fat. In these situations, you'll want to order a diet soda instead of a hot dog, a bag of licorice instead of a big tub of buttered popcorn, and fat-free tortilla chips instead of fried tortilla chips. These are better bad choices, and they are essential to your eating program. And as contrarian as this might sound, when you are between a rock and a hard place, it's still better to eat than not eat at all, even if it's a bad choice.

There are obviously going to be times when you reach certain emotional states—a terrible day at the office, for example, or even PMS—during which you will see food as a sort of solace. You'll come home at the end of the day wanting to eat fat and sugar. This is when you need to have the right kinds of bad choices in your kitchen, such as sugar-free popsicles instead of ice cream bars, dried fruit instead of candy, fat-free crackers instead of cookies, baked potato chips instead of fried, and diet soda instead of regular soda.

EATING THE LARRY NORTH WAY
The First Week

In the first week, all I want is for you to reduce caloric beverages, including alcohol, soft drinks, and fruit juice (which is basically sugar water once the fruit fiber has been removed). Replace them with milk or water. That's it! If you need to, make a list of these items on a sheet of paper and carry it with you wherever you go. Don't worry about cutting anything else out.

The other thing I want you to do is to start identifying foods you are eating that have fat—including oils, salad dressings, and fried foods. What you'll begin to realize is that you are adding massively to your fat intake in ways you don't even notice— spreading a heavy layer of butter across a slice of bread, for instance, when you'd be happy with a thin layer.

Finally, try to increase your meal frequency. Remember, nothing in the first week should feel difficult. If you are someone who has been eating poorly and needs a guideline to start, here's a sample day's menu:

Meal One: Cereal with skim milk, two whole eggs with two additional egg whites, two slices of toast with jam.

Meal Two: A turkey sandwich with mustard (never mayonnaise) and a bowl of rice.

Meal Three: For your midafternoon snack, a piece of fruit and maybe some crunchy vegetables.

Meal Four: A meat such as white fish, a potato, corn, and a salad with lemon or vinegar dressing.

Meal Five: For your evening snack, a bowl of oatmeal (little or no sugar) instead of something full of fat like ice cream.

In the first week, you can have three cheat meals. They can be anything you want. But as I've said, make sure when cheating to eat only a regular-sized meal, not a binge.

The Second Week

In the second week, in addition to what you've already cut out in the first week, I want you to cut back your dairy consumption. If you're craving dairy items, try skim milk, nonfat yogurt, or nonfat cheese. Additionally, you should totally rid your diet of all fast food. That means greasy burgers, tacos, fried chicken, and french fries. Finally, you're going to add more balance to your meals. Here's a schedule:

Meal One: Whole grain cereal (such as shredded wheat or oatmeal) with skim milk, toast with jam, and egg whites. (I'll show you how to prepare egg whites in Chapter Five.)

Meal Two: Turkey sandwich and mustard, a baked potato with salsa, nonfat yogurt, or nonfat sour cream (no butter or regular sour cream).

Meal Three: One portion of grilled chicken, a cup of rice, and a cup of fibrous vegetables, such as broccoli.

Meal Four: Baked fish, salad, and a moderate portion of pasta.

Meal Five: Fruit or crunchy vegetables for a late-night snack.

Remember that I am only giving you *examples* of food you can eat. You may choose to eat whatever protein you want, for example, as long as you select only the leanest varieties. In the second week, you are allowed to eat two cheat meals. Note there are still processed foods such as pasta and cereal in the meal plan. This is because we are making gradual changes.

The Third Week

Adding to the list of reduced food choices, in the third week I want you to reduce as much of your sugar intake as you can. That means not only soft drinks, alcohol, and desserts, but also anything with added amounts of sugar. Look for any product containing dextrose, fructose, and sucrose, or any other form of sugar from honey to syrup. We're also adding a far more balanced fifth meal.

Meal One: Five egg whites, cereal with skim milk, two slices of dry toast (notice that we have cut out the jam).

Meal Two: Grilled chicken with rice and a fibrous vegetable.

Meal Three: A meal similar to Meal Two

Meal Four: White fish, chicken, or a very lean cut of red meat (remember, cook without oil), a complex carbohydrate (potato or rice), and a salad with lemon or vinegar dressing.

Meal Five: Same as Meal One.

This week, you only get one cheat meal. But try to make it a healthier cheat than usual. If you want pizza as your cheat meal, for instance, then try it without cheese. If you want Mexican food, ask that the chips be removed from the table and replaced with corn tortillas.

The Fourth Week

You are now going to knock processed foods, such as pastas, breads, and cereal, out of the program. Try also to eat out less (so you won't be subjected to the hidden fats and oils of restaurant food), and get into the habit of healthy cooking and having food on hand so you can eat every three hours.

In this week's meal plan, pay extra attention to your balance of proteins, carbohydrates, and fibrous vegetables. Try very hard to get in all five meals.

Meal One: Four to six egg whites and one bowl of oatmeal.

Meal Two: Chicken, rice, and a fibrous vegetable.

Meal Three: A meal similar to Meal Two.

Meal Four: Meat, a complex carbohydrate, and a fibrous vegetable—similar to Meals Two and Three.

Meal Five: Same as Meal One.

The Fifth Week

Now you've reached the advanced level of the North Program. You are ready to eliminate completely those foods that you have only reduced in the previous weeks. For your meal plan, eat exactly as indicated for the fourth week.

The Sixth Week

Congratulations. If you've been following the program so far, you have seen tremendous change already. Believe it or not, you can make even more progress. Are you up for the challenge? The first step is to eliminate all cheating, to the best of your ability. Try to strip every ounce of excess fat from your diet. You'll discover in this streamlined, perfect week that your body's metabolism will fly, burning up everything in sight. You'll feel lean. You also, quite frankly, will feel hungry, so I've added a sixth meal. You won't be able to wait for that next meal. But try not to cheat under any circumstances! Remember, you only have to try this for a week. (If you are a woman, you won't require a sixth meal.)

Meal One: Oatmeal and four to six egg whites.

Meal Two: A small serving of turkey breast, a cup of rice, and a cup of broccoli.

Meal Three: Grilled chicken breast, a baked potato, a cup of corn and one fibrous vegetable.

Meal Four: Steamed fish, a serving of beans, and a salad with lemon dressing.

Meal Five: Chicken, a serving of potato, and a fibrous vegetable.

Meal Six (around 10:00 P.M.): Same as Meal One.

Do I Need A Sixth Meal?

Those of you who are really active—who are faithful about a good exercise program—will find that you're particularly ravenous, so you can add a sixth meal. You might be asking, "Why eat six meals a day? Isn't five enough?" I'm not declaring absolutely that you have to eat the sixth meal. If you're tired, not hungry, or in great need of losing weight, skip it. You won't hurt your program. But if you're flourishing on the program, and you want to continue gaining muscle, then a small sixth meal is very important. Indeed, the sixth meal is a great boost in keeping the metabolism revved up and providing the protein to build your muscle.

But Even Five Meals Seem Like a Lot for a Woman!

I know you still may not be convinced you will ever eat five meals a day, especially if you're a woman. Do this for me. As long as you believe you must eat only three meals a day, make sure those three meals are perfectly balanced and the serving sizes are correct. Eventually, as you stay with the program, you'll want a fourth meal, and then a fifth.

You may very well decide you only need minimal meals in the midmorning and midafternoon. Fine. Just make sure they are healthy and remain balanced.

Do I Have to Stay on the Sixth Week Meal Plan?

That's up to you. You should try to stay at this level of eating as long as you achieve your desired shape.

But if you do back off, don't drop to the level of the first or second week of the program. And don't think you can revert completely to bad eating habits and then come roaring right back to the level of eating I suggest for the sixth week. If you do have a major setback, it's much less difficult psychologically to ease back into the program than jump right into the intensity of the sixth week.

Still, don't feel guilty if you do lapse. We're all human, and I don't expect you to be perfect. This program is a way of life—not a class in which you pass or fail. So don't get obsessed if you have cheated, because that kind of thinking represents a dieting mentality, something I'm weaning you from. The last thing I want is for you to starve for a day or two to punish yourself for your lapse. Ultimately, that behavior will only lead to failure.

The most important result of sticking with the program through the sixth week is a more efficient metabolism, which makes small cheats okay. You'll be able to eat an extra cookie here and there, because it will get burned up in your fuel-efficient body. Just don't overdo it: If you cheat every day, those empty calories will catch up with you and reverse the results you've worked so hard for. Occasional cheating is one thing. Regular cheating is permanently falling off the program. For added fat loss, you may reduce your carb intake, but only in your final meal of the day (provided you have eaten the appropriate number of meals).

Chapter Four

EATING OUT: HOW TO STAY ON THE PROGRAM AWAY FROM HOME

It's easy to discard all the bad food in your refrigerator and pantry and bring in only good food from your neighborhood grocery store. It would be a snap to do the North Program if you could lock yourself in your house with only the leanest, healthiest foods. But that's only part of the equation. Most Americans eat away from home an average of four times a week and spend 40 percent of their monthly food budgets at restaurants. Obviously, if you

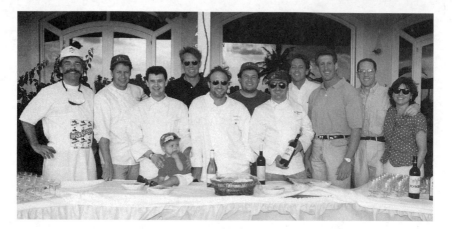

Me in the Bahamas with some of the most acclaimed
restaurant chefs in the country.

can't stay on the North Program when you're at a restaurant,
you're in trouble.

It would have been nearly impossible a decade ago to stay
on the North Program if you went to a restaurant. But the good
news today is that even some fast-food restaurants are serving
fresh salad and baked potatoes. You can find things on menus at
most restaurants that say "low-fat" or "healthy heart" or "lite." It's
not hard to find steamed or grilled vegetables and orders of lean
meat that are grilled or baked.

Still, you have to be very careful. Most restaurants continue
to serve foods with hidden fats—even those advertising "healthy"
food. Although waiters will tell you they use just a little oil on their
food, it's just as possible that the cooks in the back are drowning
the food in fat. They may marinate chicken breasts in oil or butter
or cook rice with butter and oil; vegetables are almost always
prepared in butter.

In this chapter, I'll show you how to control your meals outside your house and how to create, at any restaurant you choose,
what I like to call The North Plate.

TALKING TO YOUR WAITER

I am amazed when I see hard-driving businessmen and
businesswomen—tough negotiators at the conference table—
turn completely passive at a restaurant table. They seem to be in-

timidated by their waiters or waitresses and sometimes can't even muster the courage to ask for a different side dish to accompany their entrée. To follow the North Program, you can't afford to be a shrinking violet. You've got to be able to look your waiter in the eye and say, "Please, this is very important. Make sure my chicken is cooked in no oil or butter. I can't have it any other way." Right now, in the privacy of your own room, take a deep breath and say the following: "I cannot have any sauces on my food." There, now how hard was that?

I have one devotee of the North Program who is so determined that he says to his waiter, "Listen, I have a heart condition, and if there's any oil in my food, I could very well have cardiac arrest right here on the floor." You don't have to go that far, of course. But there's nothing wrong with letting your waiter know firmly that you want your food prepared without fat, and that if your wishes are not fulfilled adequately, you'll send it back.

Every time you go into restaurant, no matter what you order, get used to telling your waiter, "I really want to eat here, but I have a few special requests. I would like my food prepared without any oil, cooking spray, or butter." Over the years, I have become very familiar with the restaurant industry. I have been a speaker at national restaurant associations, and I have consulted for restaurateurs on all different types of cuisine. What I've discovered is that as long as you smile and act friendly, the restaurant will do its best to accommodate you. They want you to come back, so nine times out of ten, they will take care of you. But you have to ask!

KNOW WHAT YOU'RE DOING

Before you go to test your new, bold persona in a restaurant, though, you need a little bit of education. You can't go into an Italian restaurant and order a steaming plate of creamy pasta and say, "And make that low in fat." No chef can take the cheese out of fettuccine Alfredo.

The waiter will respect your request more if you ask for pasta dressed only in tomato, basil, and garlic, or perhaps with a little wine. When you order fish or chicken, ask that it be cooked with lemon or lime juice as an alternative to oil or butter. Don't be shy about sending it back if it shows up swimming in oil.

Here's another common mistake. You sit down for breakfast in a restaurant and proudly ask for an egg white omelet. But you don't specify how you want it prepared. You'll get your egg whites, all right, but the omelet may be cooked in butter and covered with cheese. You end up with a thirty-fat-gram omelet! The lesson? Be specific. If you ask for an egg white omelet without cheese and prepared with no butter or oil, you bring the fat content down to zero. If you become a strict adherent to the program, you will never feel worse than when you order what you think is a low-fat piece of grilled chicken and learn later that it is swamped with fat, all because the cook added four to five tablespoons of cooking oil. As you gain experience, you'll be able to spot—and taste—the difference.

OTHER SUGGESTIONS

Here are more suggestions for eating out in restaurants:

1. Ask for vegetables that are steamed, boiled, or blanched quickly in a bit of water only.

2. Don't order any soups that have cream or meat bases. That's usually an indication of high fat.

3. Ask the waiter if the chef blanches the food in oil. That's a process in which the chef (frequently at Chinese restaurants) puts vegetables into scalding high-fat oil to cleanse or loosen the peel. Tell the waiter you do not want your food blanched in oil.

4. Ask for all dressings and sauces on the side or request that they be omitted from your order altogether. If you do use them for flavoring, dip your fork in the dressing and then spear your food. That gives you enough of a taste. Don't do it the other way around, that is, don't spear your food first and then dip it in the dressing. In that case, it will be slathered with dressing. Lemon and vinegar are great substitutes for salad dressing.

5. Ask that any nuts and seeds be removed from your dishes.

6. Ask the waiter to remove any temptations from your table, such as butter, bread, crackers, and chips. A pre-meal roll with butter is an estimated 150 calories.

7. Be careful at salad bars. Many offer high-fat choices such as bacon bits, cheese, and croutons. Avoid all prepared salads, like pasta and potato salads. They are loaded with mayonnaise and other fat contributors.

8. Avoid drinking alcohol with your meal, as it will enhance your appetite. If you do want a drink, try a wine spritzer (wine with soda), which has fewer calories than a glass of wine. Even if you drink a beer with no fat, the beer, loaded with sugar and calories, cuts down on your body's ability to burn fat.

9. Ask about side dishes that come with your meal. For example, if you order a turkey sandwich with mustard—a good choice—it may come on a plate heaped with potato chips and cole slaw, which you'll be tempted to dig into too. Tell your waiter to serve your entrée without the fattening sides.

10. Avoid the classic "Dieter's Plate" at restaurants. Although you may think it's a good choice, a typical sirloin patty, cottage cheese, and a tomato slice can be 70 percent fat.

11. Don't feel you must eat everything just because you paid for it. Remember that you usually get larger portions at a restaurant than you'd give yourself at home. Don't hesitate to share your food. Just be careful not to let your fellow diners talk you into sharing dessert. Don't be intimidated. Ask for their encouragement and tell them how great you feel since you've been on the program, and they'll stop pressuring you—and probably think twice about that dessert themselves!

MAKING A NORTH PLATE

In my hometown of Dallas, the North Plate has become a popular meal at many restaurants. It usually consists of a grilled chicken breast, brown rice, and broccoli, but you can put the same ingredients together at any restaurant, even the greasiest hamburger joint.

Always remember that at each meal you should choose a protein, a complex carbohydrate, and often a fibrous vegetable. Look the menu over very carefully to see what foods the restaurant has available. Let's take a burger restaurant. It should have lots of lettuce and tomato to dress up the hamburger. All right, there's your fibrous vegetable. They make french fries from potatoes, so ask very politely if they might have an extra baked potato lying around that you can have served plain. Okay, you've got your carb. And almost always, there's a chicken sandwich on the menu. If the chicken can be grilled without oil, get it plain (no bread, no mayonnaise), then pull off any of the skin or fat when it arrives. There's your protein.

I am convinced that if given the chance, people will usually pick a meal that is stripped of fat, as long as it's tasty.

OTHER RESTAURANTS

I know some people who don't even look at a menu when they walk into a restaurant, because they don't want to be tempted. They ask for a grilled meat, a potato dish, and a steamed vegetable. In fact, regardless of what kind of restaurant you visit, there are always specific dishes you can ask for.

French: You can ask for an egg white omelet, fillet of sole, poached sea bass, trout, bay scallops, or other grilled fish or white meat in wine sauce. There's usually a standard salad you can get without dressing. If it's a spinach salad, ask that no bacon or egg be added. Avoid hollandaise or any cream-based sauce, as well as sautéed dishes. Avoid high-fat dishes such as duck, pâté, and foie gras.

Italian: Look for a vegetable plate with no sauce, meatless pasta with oil-free marinara or wine sauce, or a vegetarian pizza with no cheese and an oil-free crust. Avoid cream sauces and fatty foods such as prosciutto, Parmesan cheese, breaded veal, breaded vegetables, and white breads. Also watch out for olive oil, which many restaurants tend to overuse. Plain pasta might seem to be a good choice, but it often contains oil from the water in which it is boiled. One of my favorite Italian meals consists of grilled portabello mushrooms with balsamic vinegar, grilled chicken Caesar salad with no croutons (dressing on the side), and a small bowl of plain pasta (marinara sauce on the side). When I make it, I can make sure there's no oil in it.

Mexican: Look for fresh fish or chicken breast marinated in lime sauce with beans and rice. You can also order unfried corn tortillas, chicken enchiladas without the cheese or cream sauce, or chicken fajitas grilled in lemon or lime juice instead of oil. Avoid cheese, chips, sour cream, guacamole, and refried beans (ask for whole beans instead). It's easy to make a North Plate at a Mexican restaurant: Just order grilled chicken fajitas with no oil, corn tortillas (instead of higher fat flour tortillas), rice instead of refried beans, pico de gallo instead of guacamole, and no cheese. Have the lettuce, onion, and tomato on the side. If you see spinach enchiladas on the menu, you can ask for a side of steamed spinach as your fibrous vegetable.

Chinese: Go for Moo Goo Gai Pan without sauce. Ask for fresh or steamed fish and vegetables. Make sure only white meat chicken is used in dishes. Ask that the dishes be stir-fried in broth or water instead of oil or salt. Choose dishes that come with sliced meat rather than diced meat, because diced meat is often from fattier cuts. Order steamed rice instead of fried rice. Avoid egg rolls, any batter-fried item, any egg dishes, and dishes loaded with nuts. Don't order beef or pork, and never order the duck (an average three-and-a-half ounce serving of Peking duck has 30 grams of fat).

Vietnamese, Thai, or Japanese: These restaurants are great for the North Program, because they often use very little oil in their cooking. You can order any type of dish with no egg and no oil, and it's likely to be low in fat. You can also order a spring roll that's like an egg roll, but make sure it is not fried. Japanese restaurants also cook many items without oil or margarine. Sushi places can be ideal for your program, as long as you order the less fattening items on the menu. I recommend the California roll minus the avocado and mayonnaise. However, be careful, because some sushi, such as eel and ahi tuna, can be extremely high in fat, and of course avoid anything that is fried.

Indian: You can find low-fat legumes, steamed vegetables, chicken, and fish that has been marinated and roasted without oil on many Indian restaurant menus. Chutney condiments add a lot of flavor without adding fat. But don't overdo them. Chutney still contains a lot of sugar.

Steak house: At a steak restaurant, ask for a large dinner salad without cheese or croutons and a baked potato with yogurt or Dijon mustard. Most of these restaurants also offer grilled chicken. If you go with chicken, ask that all fat be trimmed and no oil be used in preparation. You can usually have shrimp or perhaps lobster. But if you went there to eat steak, then order one. My suggestion is to get a smaller cut (six ounces is a good size) of filet mignon and have the chef butterfly it on the grill, a process in which he cuts it down the middle (this way, some of the fat drains out in the grilling process).

Fast Food: There is very little nutritional value in fast food. It hits you with a horde of sugar and fat calories without any fiber or vitamins. And don't be fooled into thinking that fast-food chicken is better than a hamburger. A single fried chicken nugget contains an entire tablespoon of mostly saturated fat, and fast-food chicken sandwiches have as much fat as hamburgers. As for fried chicken, the originally healthy piece is so soaked in oil that the fat has seeped down to the bone. If you must eat at a fast-food restaurant, try to go vegetarian. Get the lettuce and tomato and look for a baked potato.

Pizza place: At a pizza restaurant, order a pizza with peppers, mushrooms, onions, shrimp, and chicken, if available— and no cheese. That alone saves you a tremendous number of calories. If you want a little additional flavor, you can add a bit of extra sauce.

American chain restaurants: Actually, these restaurants have become very acceptable for North eaters. Most of them carry grilled chicken, grilled shrimp, brown rice, black beans, salads, fat-free dressing, and steamed vegetables.

Cafeterias: Again, at cafeterias, turn to salads. Most of the meats offered at cafeterias are soaked in oil or butter, as are the vegetables. Your safest choices are going to be straight dinner salads with dressing on the side. Avoid all casseroles, and ask how the vegetables have been cooked.

Greasy Spoon: You can even follow the North Program here. If you're eating breakfast, try five to seven hard-boiled or poached egg whites, a bowl of oatmeal, and dry toast. Sometimes you can special-order a grilled white meat item and vegetables that are not sautéed, fried, or buttered.

Fine Dining: In all likelihood, there will be times in your life when you'll be at special occasion or five-star restaurants, and those will be times when you just don't want to special-order. Great. Go for it. I've always believed that if you're going to cheat, you should make every bite count. The only thing I would do at such restaurants is order your sauces on the side instead of letting the chef coat your food with them. Also be careful with the vegetables, because they are usually soaking in butter.

EATING WHILE TRAVELING

There will be times when you are out of town and can't find a restaurant to serve your needs. On those occasions, it's just as convenient to stop at a local grocery store or deli and get four to five ounces of sliced, salt-free turkey, order a baked potato, buy some carrots and a green apple—and there's your meal!

If you are traveling by airplane, you can order a special meal or prepare a small container or cooler of food, including fresh sliced or canned turkey or chicken, raw vegetables, and a piece of fruit. At your hotel, you can ask the manager or the concierge to honor your requests. (They'll even get you a portable microwave or a small refrigerator to store a healthy meal or two, so you don't have to go through the hassle of looking for an accommodating restaurant.) There are plenty of ways to be creative on the North Program. All you need is the desire to do it.

MEAL REPLACEMENT PRODUCTS

Protein powders and protein drinks have been around for decades. In the past, you've had to hold your nose to get them down your throat, and the quality of protein has been very dubious. But today, as a result of better technology, these protein powders and meal replacement products are packaged in premeasured quantities. Many of them are low in sugar and offer relatively adequate quantities of protein and carbs.

I have no objection to most of them. They mix well with water, so you can use them anywhere. Just shake them in a shaker or mix them in a blender. They're particularly convenient for those times when you simply cannot have an adequate meal. Moreover, if you get tired of eating so much protein during the day, the protein substitute in powder form serves as a nice alternative to egg whites and chicken.

But be careful. There are still companies overloading their meal replacement products with sugar to get them to taste better. Even more dangerous, you may be tempted to improve the flavor of the concoction with your own ingredients, like ice cream, whole milk, or fruit juice. Don't do it! And don't consider meal replacement products some kind of miracle food. They should be at most an occasional meal substitute. Because they lack fiber and don't stop food cravings (only real food helps you deal with your craving for food), you should never make them a staple of your program.

If you want to try one of these products, look on the back of the package to make sure there is an adequate distribution of proteins and carbs (Met-Rx, RX Fuel, Designer Protein, and EAS are good brands), and be sure that there is no hidden sugar.

STAY FOCUSED

Many of you will finish this chapter and think, "Well, it seems so troublesome to have to special-order every single time I walk into a restaurant." Or, "Larry has made good points, but I'm sure I'll get some benefit if I do a little bit of the program, like ordering salad dressing on the side or more grilled chicken."

Yes, you'll see some results. You won't get any fatter, for one. But you won't get really lean unless you make a real commitment to ordering the North way.

Initially, I admit, it does seem like a hassle to give your speech to the waiter about special-ordering. But it's no different from being a kid learning to say "Yes, sir" and "No, sir" to an adult. Once you get in the habit, you don't even think twice about it anymore.

That's exactly the way I am when I special-order. If I'm eating with someone for the first time, he or she will look at me and say, "You do that every time?" I look back and say, "Do what every time?" I don't even think about it, because it's second nature.

If you get weary of special-ordering, think about this. The fifteen extra seconds you spend telling the waiter what you want at each meal could save you 1,500 calories by the end of the day. To me, that's worth your time.

■ THE I DON'T KNOW HOW TO COOK BOOK: LARRY'S FOOD LOVER'S GUIDE TO COOKING

■ I know you're laughing. Someone like me teaching you to cook? Isn't that about the same as Martha Stewart teaching you to lift weights?

The fact is that there are a lot of people—even in this highly food-conscious age—who don't have a clue how to prepare some basic meals: how to crack open an egg or make grilled chicken or brown rice. There are plenty of men who are too intimidated to turn on a stove, and just as many women who have been so busy conducting the rest of their lives that they have never taken the time to learn how to cook well.

The good news, however, is that healthy low-fat cooking has never been easier. It's not time-consuming, and it doesn't take extra effort or a trained gourmet chef's touch. Nevertheless, there's no question that you need to be reminded of some basic things that will help you prepare the right foods. If you don't have those at your fingertips, then it's going to be hard to stay on the North eating program.

Right here, I'd like to give all the credit to what you're about to read to my wife, Melanie North, who in 1990 started what is now a wildly popular Dallas catering company, Good Square Meals, which specializes in great-tasting nonfat meals. Mel is also the brains behind the concept of and recipes for our first restaurant, North-South. As a customer at North-South, if you want a certain dish prepared with no oil, no butter, and sauce on the side, you tell the waiter you want it prepared the "North" way. If you want a regularly prepared meal, you tell the waiter you want it the "South" way.

THE BASIC KITCHEN

In preparing meals suggested in this book, a microwave is very helpful to save time, while a grill enhances the taste of your food. Grills also save time, because there is far less cleanup required.

To follow this program, you need significant freezer space, because ideally you will be cooking in quantity. Consider buying a second-hand upright freezer to put in your garage or basement. If you are single and live alone, the freezer in your refrigerator will probably be fine.

When it comes to a stove, if you have a choice, choose gas. It saves you time, because it heats up and cools down more quickly. Another advantage of gas is that it's easy to keep on very low settings, which is helpful when cooking with low-fat and nonfat cheeses. Ideally, you want a gas stove and an electric broiler because the temperature control is more consistent on electric broilers. If gas is not an option for you, don't worry. You can prepare a perfectly good meal on an electric stove. You can even "grill" without a grill. Look for the new ridged grill pans found in any specialty cooking store.

Utensil and Appliance Musts

Food processor: You don't need a complicated food processor with a ton of options. Just buy a mini food processor with one speed, a chopping blade, and a powerful motor. When you shop, look for ease of operation.

Hand blender: Okay, they do use these a lot on the gourmet cooking shows, but don't be intimidated—they are great for making shakes and thickening soups.

Nonstick skillet: There are two schools of thought here. Either buy a really cheap $3 skillet at the grocery store and replace it every couple of months when the finish begins to get sticky, or buy a really good one. If you choose the latter, you'll have to spend quite a lot more for one; it will last a long time if you take care of it, just following these rules: Never put it in the dishwasher; never heat it past medium high when it's empty; never use metal utensils on the surface; never scrub it with a scrubbing pad (use a regular sponge and hot soapy water); and never use nonstick cooking spray in it, which will gum up the surface. Before cooking, just rub some butter or oil directly on it with a paper towel, or spray it with water or chicken broth from a spray bottle. (Scanpan is one brand on which you can use metal utensils and scrub sponges. I've found them great for everything but omelets.)

Knives: It's important to have sharp, good quality knives. Look for a German make. You'll need at least one serrated and one nonserrated.

Pots and pans: You really only need as many pots and pans as you have burners.

Pyrex: Buy one Pyrex pan for lasagne.

Cookie sheet: Buy one basic cookie sheet. It doesn't have to be nonstick, because you can cover it with foil before use.

Mixing bowls: You'll need several sizes.

Pot holders: Don't grab hot things with your bare hands!

Aluminum foil: Foil saves you hours in cleanup time.

Timers: Have several kitchen timers on hand, so you can cook several things at once.

Measuring spoons and cups: It's fine to use a pinch of this and a dash of that, but you'll also need these.

Cutting board: Buy a Sanatec or a wooden one, because the Sanatec can be put in the dishwasher and the wood has antibacterial properties that help you keep a healthy kitchen. Neither one will damage your knives as can glass, hard plastic, or marble.

Vegetable peeler: Don't just settle for the one from the grocery store. It really makes a difference if you have a good, sharp one, and that means you'll have to pay more than $1.99 for it.

Cooking utensils: If you buy only plastic or wood cooking utensils—basically spoons and spatulas—then you won't have to worry about ruining your nonstick pan with metal ones. However, you will need a few metal utensils—tongs and a spatula with a longer handle—for grilling.

Wire cooling rack: Even though it's called a cooling rack, you'll be using this to bake.

Colander: For draining pasta and washing salad lettuces.

Grater: This will come in handy for cheese and for other ingredients when you don't need enough to warrant getting out your food processor.

Kitchen shears: Cooking scissors that are great for trimming chicken, snipping herbs, and much, much more.

Storage containers: Buy plenty of freezer-to-microwave containers—some divided for individual meals and others large enough for multiple portions of one thing, like mashed potatoes.

Freezer zip bags: You'll use these for marinating and food storage.

Apron: You may feel like the Galloping Gourmet, but if you wear one, you'll save on your cleaning bill.

Sponges: Buy these often. Don't keep the same one for a year and let it turn black. Put them in the dishwasher for easy sanitization.

Plastic wrap: To cover food when it's being stored temporarily.

TV: To keep you company if you cook alone and to entice you to cook while watching your favorite shows. Instead of blowing off cooking, you can do both at once.

Basic Everyday Dishes

In the appendix of this book, you will find Melanie's best no-added-fat recipes—recipes you will be able to prepare after you finish this chapter. You'll find it's not difficult to cook, once you begin, but you may need instructions on how to prepare some basic meals to start you on your way. What I'm going to do now is take you through a day of low-fat meals, with specific guidance on cooking healthy, low-fat dishes on the North Program.

Morning Foods

1. *Oatmeal:* I suggest using three-minute oatmeal because it tastes better. You can eat it dry or with skim milk, or pour boiling water over it. Another quick-prep involves mixing the oatmeal with tap water in a bowl and microwaving it for a minute and a half. Eat it with such extras as cinnamon, Butter Buds, nutmeg, or berries.

2. *Hard-boiled eggs:* Bring water in a pot to a boil, gently drop in the eggs, and boil for 10 to 15 minutes. Alternatively, set the eggs in the water, bring to a boil, turn off the heat, and let sit for 20 minutes. This method saves energy. Here's a secret to peeling eggs, which few people do well. As soon as you pull a hot egg from the pot, hold it

under cold running water while you peel. Of course, eat only the egg whites.

3. *Scrambled egg whites:* Crack the egg gently in half, but let nothing run out. Now you face the task of getting the egg white out while keeping the yolk in the shell. Holding the two halves of the cracked egg, pour the egg yolk from shell to shell and let all the egg white drip into a bowl. Discard the yolk. Repeat for as many eggs as you need. Pour the egg whites into a preheated nonstick skillet. Scramble the whites with a wooden, plastic, or rubber utensil (using a metal utensil with nonstick cookware will ruin the cookware).

4. *Egg-white omelet:* Separate the eggs and set aside the bowl of whites. Chop desired ingredients (onions, green pepper, tomatoes, cooked chicken breast, broccoli, for instance) and either precook them in the microwave or on the stove (cooking the ingredients in water only, no oils or butter). Reserve. Pour your egg whites into a skillet on a low setting, but do not scramble. When the whites begin to set, take a wooden spoon and gently make small incisions about an inch long in your omelet so the uncooked parts of the egg whites can flow into the bottom of the skillet. When most of the whites are cooked, cover the skillet. The steam will cook the remainder. Uncover and gently loosen the entire perimeter of the omelet from the pan with a plastic spatula. Turn the heat off. Pour on your drained vegetable and/or chicken ingredients, then gently fold the omelet in half, still keeping it in the skillet. Now, you must act like a real chef. Slide the omelet out of the skillet onto the plate, shout "Voilà!" in a French accent, and there you have it. If you mess up and break the omelet, then just mix it around in the skillet and you have—voilà again!—scrambled eggs.

Chicken, Fish, and Meat

Make sure, whatever meat you get, to trim off the skin and all visible fat before cooking.

1. *Baked chicken* or *fish:* Cover a baking sheet with foil and preheat the oven to 350 degrees. Place skinless chicken breast or fish on the sheet, season it, then bake it: for chicken 20 to 25 minutes, for fish 10 minutes per inch of thickness, measure the thickest part. For a variation on taste, marinate and dredge lightly in breadcrumbs.

2. *Poached chicken* or *fish:* Put herbs and one cup of wine (you can also add Dijon mustard or lemon juice) into a skillet. Place chicken or fish in skillet, cover, and simmer on low heat for 10 minutes for fish, for chicken 20 minutes.

3. *Grilled chicken, fish, or lean cuts of beef:* Marinate your meat in any variety of nonfat liquids—nonfat chicken broth with spices, any sort of citrus juices, fat-free barbecue sauce, or low-sodium soy sauce with ginger and garlic—then slap the chicken, beef, or pork on the grill for 7 to 10 minutes on each side. For fish cook only for a total of 10 minutes per inch, 5 minutes each side. Don't try to poke the meat with a knife, because it will release all the meat's juices.

4. *Broiled chicken* or *fish* or *lean cuts of meat (beef or pork):* Preheat the broiler, cover a baking sheet with foil, season your chicken or fish, and broil. This type of cooking is very fast, about 5 minutes or less a side, for fish, and 20 minutes total, 10 minutes each side for chicken or lean cuts of meat, so after a few minutes, check to see if the meat is done, then flip it over to complete the other side.

5. *Turkey breast:* Put a turkey breast with desired seasonings in a foil cooking bag and bake in the oven at 325 degrees. Cook for 20 minutes a pound.

6. *Microwaved fish:* Buy a white fish fillet, rinse it, sprinkle dill, parsley, and/or lemon pepper over it, and add the juice of half a lemon. Place the fish on a plate, cover with plastic wrap, pop it in the microwave for a couple of minutes, and serve. Remarkably tasty.

7. *Tuna salad:* To make a delicious tuna salad, start with waterpacked tuna and fat-free mayonnaise. Put in onion, celery, and egg whites. If you're an adventurous eater, add Dijon mustard, vinegar, cilantro, tomatoes, and onion.

Vegetables

1. *Dried beans:* Rinse dried beans in a strainer. Pour the beans into a bowl four times bigger than the amount of the beans (to allow for expansion), cover with water, and let stand overnight. The next day, dump out the water, rinse the beans again, put them in a pot filled with fresh water, and bring them to a boil for 10 minutes. Let them cool completely, drain the water again (this is the best technique to avoid digestive gas), rinse, fill the pot again with fresh water to cover, and bring to a boil, then turn the heat down to a simmer. Simmer for 1 to 2 hours until the beans are soft. You can add seasoning such as liquid smoke, garlic, and onion. If you're adventurous, experiment with herbs like basil, oregano, chili powder, and red pepper.

2. *Broccoli:* Cut off the stalks of the broccoli and peel. Skinned broccoli stems are the most tasty and nutritious part. Put the broccoli stems and florets on a plate, wrap in plastic, and microwave for 2 minutes or until the broccoli turns bright green. (For best results, make sure the broccoli stems are facing the walls of the microwave.) Alternatively, put the broccoli in a skillet with water and cover with a collapsible steamer. Cook over high heat for 10 to 20 minutes. Don't use too much water, or the vitamins will leach away. Finally, you can stir-fry broccoli by breaking the bunch into bite-sized pieces, chopping up a couple of cloves of garlic, and stirring them together on medium heat—you can add a little water or broth for moisture—until the broccoli turns bright green.

3. *Corn on the cob:* If you buy your corn still in the husk, remove husks and silk by peeling back and snapping off at the base of the ear. Wash in running water to com-

pletely remove corn silk. Cook the same as broccoli or boil in a big pot of water for 5 minutes. Use Molly McButter or Butter Buds, but put on the butter substitutes while the corn is still steaming hot. It will taste better. Of course, never slather on any real butter!

4. *Carrots:* Slice into coin-sized pieces, drop in a pot of water, and cook for 10 to 15 minutes. For extra flavor, add a tablespoon of maple syrup for each carrot.

5. *Brown rice:* Bring a pot of water to a boil and drop in the rice. (For every cup of rice, you need two cups of water.) Cover the pot and leave it on simmer for 45 minutes. You can cook in chicken broth instead of water for a taste variation, or add a package of chicken noodle soup. You can also try adding diced onions, bell peppers, cilantro, mushrooms, onions, or white wine.

6. *Baking potatoes:* Buy russet potatoes for baking. Preheat oven to 450 degrees, pierce the potatoes a couple of times with a fork, then bake for 45 minutes. If you bake your potatoes without foil, they'll come out a little more fluffy. Microwaving your potatoes takes 8 to 10 minutes! Your potato won't be as fluffy or have a crispy skin, but you won't heat up your kitchen either. Instead of butter, margarine, or sour cream for toppings, try salsa, nonfat yogurt, nonfat butter substitutes, and chives. Want to try Larry's Loaded Baked Potato? After you've baked your potato, take deli-sliced turkey, wrap it in a paper towel, and pop it into the microwave on high for a few minutes. Then crumble the turkey, which now tastes like bacon bits, over the potato and add a butter substitute, or nonfat topping. C'est magnifique!

7. *New potatoes:* Cut your new potatoes into chunks, put them in a pot of water, and boil at high or medium for 20 minutes or until soft. They're ready to serve, or you can use them to create a potato salad using nonfat mayonnaise, green onion, pepper, and dill.

8. *Larry Fries:* After microwaving, boiling, or baking a potato (the potato does not have to be fully cooked),

shave it into thin pieces. Cover a cookie sheet with foil and lay out the pieces. Sprinkle the potato slices with seasonings like garlic powder, paprika, salt, and pepper. Broil the potato slices until brown and puffy on one side. Flip them over with a spatula. Broil the second side. Pull out perfect, nonfat fries.

9. *Tossed salad:* Use a combination of lettuces, shred carrots in a grater, slice a bell pepper, and toss in any other fresh raw vegetables you want. For a new kind of low-fat dressing, buy a vinaigrette, pour out all the oil (that settles on the top before shaking), and use what's left. Or try vinegar and Dijon mustard mixed with honey.

Remember, these are just some suggestions for elementary dishes. Turn to page 000 in the Appendix for a six-week plan of fantastic, sophisticated meals that will never be boring.

Supplies

To have the right ingredients on hand when you're ready to cook, put these things in your pantry:

Tomato sauce, canned whole tomatoes, crushed tomatoes

Chicken broth and beef broth

Balsamic vinegar

Red or white wine vinegar

Rice wine vinegar (it's smoother in salad dressings and great for Chinese food)

Evaporated skim milk

White wine, sherry, and red wine

Cornstarch

Flour

Sweetener, either sugar or a substitute (remember, you can't cook with Equal but you can cook with Sweet 'n' Low)

Butter Buds

Bread crumbs

Instant soups—not canned, but the powders you add hot
water to (most are low in fat, but read the label to make
sure); these are great when you are really hungry and
need something immediately

Lipton onion soup mix

Chicken bouillon

Jar of spaghetti sauce and pasta—these never go bad and
can always be heated for a quick meal

Brown rice and rice mixes

Oatmeal

Canned beans (take less time to prepare than dried beans)

Canned mushrooms

Boxed cereal (choose something like Cheerios or shredded
wheat that has at least some nutritive value)

Canned tuna fish

Cocoa powder

Baking powder

Baking soda

Onions and potatoes

Put these things in your refrigerator:

Olive oil or other vegetable oil

Ketchup

Barbecue sauce

Soy sauce

Worcestershire sauce

Jar of chopped garlic

Mustards

Hot sauces

Fat-free mayonnaise

Fat-free salad dressings

Nonfat milk

Chutneys

Capers

Prepared sauces (make sure to read the labels and only buy low-fat or nonfat varieties only)

Pickles

Salsa

Eggs

Baby carrots, prewashed

Salad (in a bag for convenience)

Fresh broccoli

Corn in season

Green peppers

Berries

Apples, preferably Granny Smith, because they're lower in sugar

Nonfat cheeses

Nonfat sour cream

Sugar-free Jell-O

Put these things in your freezer:

Turkey bacon (that you make yourself by dehydrating turkey breast in the microwave; see page 200 in the appendix for the method)

Ice cube trays of frozen broth, sauce, or any other useful left-over liquids. After they are frozen, take them out and transfer them to zipper bags for storage.

Grated fresh ginger—store in a zipper bag squeezed flat to remove air and get at the amount you need

Frozen green beans

Frozen peas

Frozen corn

Frozen chopped spinach—buy a name brand instead of a store brand to avoid getting too many stems

Vegetable mixtures for quick stir-fries (check the sauces in the packages for fat content before using them)

Frozen hash browns

Chicken breasts

Sliced Canadian bacon

Frozen berries—the quality is always consistent and the frozen varieties don't suffer from seasonality of prices

Popsicles

Your own frozen dinners

Herbs and Spices

What's the difference, you ask? Herbs more closely resemble the plants they came from. Think leaves. Spices are spicy, zesty, aromatic, and usually ground down to powders (take cinnamon, for example). Store your dried herbs and spices in a cool, dark, dry place. A good rule of thumb for taste testing is that if they change color after you buy them, they have changed taste. Your dried oregano (not ground) is green when you buy it; it should be green when you use it. After a year, check your herbs and spices for color or changes in aroma. You might want to check paprika more frequently, because it has a tendency to get buggy.

Crush dried herbs between your fingers when adding to food to release the flavor. Experiment with them: First use them in the quantity indicated in a recipe, then make changes trying different amounts or variations, noting them in the recipe. Herbs weaken in flavor when frozen, while spices intensify. Herbs can also become bitter if overcooked.

Basic herbs and spices to have on hand:

Salt and pepper

Basil

Bay leaves

Chili powder

Cinnamon

Cumin

Italian herb blend

Oregano

Paprika

Granulated garlic

Granulated onion

Rosemary
Tarragon
Dill
Thyme
Crushed red pepper

Seasonings Typical to Cuisines

Chinese

garlic
soy
ginger
Chinese five spice
star anise
rice wine vinegar
dry sherry
oyster sauce
sesame oil

Italian

oregano
basil
bay leaves
garlic
rosemary
thyme
fennel
nutmeg

Indian

cumin/cumin seed
fenugreek
garam masala (spice mixture)
turmeric

cardamom
cinnamon
cloves
curry powder (spice mixture)

Mexican

chili powder
oregano
cumin/cumin seed
cilantro
hot peppers
garlic
coriander

French

tarragon
marjoram
thyme
rosemary
bouquet garni (herb mixture)
herbes de Provence (herb mixture)
dill
saffron

Thai

garlic	mint
ginger	shrimp paste
fish sauce	soy sauce
Kaffir lime leaves (lime zest)	basil
lemongrass	chili paste/hot pepper
cilantro	

STORING FOOD—OR HOW TO AVOID FOOD POISONING

Actually, nothing in your freezer should go bad, except for some fatty fishes, which can turn rancid. But after a certain time, taste, texture, and nutritive values are lost from frozen foods. Following are some guidelines for how long you can keep something in the freezer or refrigerator and expect it to taste right.

- Freeze any liquid in ice cube trays, then put cubes in freezer bags and they'll last 4 to 6 months.

- Meals in freezer containers also last 4 to 6 months.

- Leftovers stored properly—in an airtight container or covered—in the refrigerator will last 3 to 5 days.

Specific Foods

- Poultry—9 months in the freezer

- Beef—6 to 12 months in the freezer

- Pork—4 to 6 months in the freezer

- Fish—6 to 8 months in the freezer

- Milk products—a month in the freezer, a week after opening in the refrigerator. Sour cream and cheese will last longer than a month if they aren't contaminated by a used utensil, dirty hands, or your mouth. Watch for mold or scum, and if an item smells bad, dump it.

- Whole eggs—3 weeks if uncooked, a week if cooked, in the refrigerator

- Uncooked egg whites—a week in the refrigerator. You can also freeze egg whites. Put 6 in a zipper bag, and they'll keep for several months.

- Syrups and honey—more than a year in the pantry

- Condiments in general—anything with salt, sugar, or vinegar has the benefit of natural preservative and will probably last until you run out of it, but let taste be your guide.

- Ketchup, Worcestershire, hot pepper sauce—6 months or more in the refrigerator

- Mustard—2 years in the refrigerator

- Mayonnaise—this is not as dangerous as was once thought. Let your eyes and nose be your guide. If it smells or tastes bad, dump it.

- Oil—tends to go rancid in about 6 months, but if it smells and tastes okay, it's still good.

More Preservation Guidelines

Here are more guidelines on preserving food: Soft foods with any mold on them should be thrown away. That goes for cucumbers, lettuce, berries, peaches, melons, breads, cakes, rolls, and flour. Ditto for sliced or shredded cheeses, yogurt, nonfat dairy spreads and dressings, meats, canned foods, peanut butter, any kind of juice, and cooked or leftover food.

There are some things you can get away with eating after trimming the mold. These include bell peppers, broccoli, cauliflower, garlic, onions, potatoes, winter squash, apples, pears, and ungrated Parmesan, Cheddar and other hard cheeses. To use these, trim an inch away from the mold. When in doubt, toss.

Making Food Last Longer

To be safe and keep your food longer, don't stick used or otherwise contaminated utensils or your fingers in the container. Always cover or contain your food in the refrigerator.

Keep uncooked eggs in the carton—not in the tray that's in your refrigerator. Also, store them tip (or small side) down. This trick also works for yogurt and cottage cheese. If you store these upside down, they will last much longer.

Don't keep your milk in the refrigerator door. Instead, put it toward the back away from light and temperature changes.

Don't wash your produce before putting it away. If it goes into the fridge wet, it will liquefy and turn to slime. Cool and dry is what you're after. Do take your produce out of plastic bags, which can trap moisture, and do use your crisper—that's what it's there for.

A Final Note on Safety

Clean your cutting boards and counters using two teaspoons of bleach per quart of water to kill bacteria.

HOW TO READ AND USE RECIPES

Before you begin to cook, read the recipe all the way through and make sure you have everything on hand in the quantities you need to make the dish. Get everything out that you are going to need. It's often easier to do all of your chopping before you start cooking, but if you are cooking multiple recipes, sometimes it's not the most efficient way to do things. You may have waiting time while something simmers or marinates, for instance, and you can spend that time chopping. Also, look at the recipes you're going to prepare and see if you can chop common ingredients together and then divide into the specified amounts per recipe.

Definitions

mince—this means chopping into teeny tiny pieces. Do it in the food processor.

dice—the next size up from mince, ¼ inch or smaller

chop—slightly bigger, up to ½ inch. An easy way to chop herbs is to put them in a glass jar and snip them with your scissors pointed down into the bottom.

julienne—long, thin strips like toothpicks. Make thin slices lengthwise, then stack them and slice along the perpendicular.

shred—finer strips than julienne. Use the grater.

boil—cook in water. Cover what you're boiling completely with water.

broil—heat from above. Always preheat your broiler. Crack the oven door if your broiler is electric, close it if it's gas. I prefer to broil on a foil-covered cookie sheet, because cleanup is faster.

sauté—using a small amount of liquid, cook on top of the stove in a shallow pan, the strict definition would of course require a small amount of butter, fat or oil; however, this is the lowfat way to sauté.

roast—cook dry in the oven

braise—similar to roast but with liquid. Usually something braised is seared first.

sear—brown on high heat on top of the stove

stew—similar to braise but with more liquid

bake—cook in the oven

stir-fry—basically the same as sautéing. You don't need a wok to do this. You can use your nonstick pan.

deglaze—to remove the caramelized food from the bottom of the pan with a liquid like wine or broth. This method is the basis for many sauces and gravies.

poach—bring a liquid to a boil, put food in, and remove from heat *steam*—cook with water on the verge of evaporating. Water boiling below steamer should not touch food. Put a top on your pan to trap the steam.

Adapting Recipes

Following these simple guidelines, you can adapt most of your favorite recipes to be lower in fat and healthier without sacrificing taste.

Any time you see "one whole chicken" or "chicken parts," think: boneless, skinless chicken or turkey breast. One whole chicken equals six boneless, skinless breasts.

For beef, use eye of round, bottom round, or top round instead of other cuts suggested in the recipe.

Ground beef: use 90 to 95 percent lean.

Ground turkey or chicken—make sure it's breast instead of mixed parts.

For pork, use tenderloin instead of chops or pork loin roast. If your recipe calls for a pork chop, cut a 2½-inch slice of pork tenderloin and butterfly (slice almost all the way through the middle, then toward each side and spread apart) or pound it out thin.

Sautéing—Whenever a recipe calls for sautéing in any kind of fat, substitute defatted chicken broth. To defat the broth, skim the visible fat off with a spoon or paper towel.

Browning—Heat up your pan on medium-high, then pour in two tablespoons of defatted broth and let it evaporate completely. When the broth starts to brown on the pan, add whatever you need to brown, making sure you don't add too much at one time. Let it sit for a minute or two, and if your broth starts to burn, add some more broth. Don't drown it: you're not boiling. Stir only slightly. The key to this process is not moving your food around too much and not adding too much broth at once.

Dairy adaptations: Any time a recipe calls for a dairy product like cream or whole milk, use evaporated skim milk from a can or skim milk. Any time it calls for whole eggs, use two egg whites. You can't adapt any recipe that calls for separated eggs and uses only the yolks, so find something else that can be adapted.

Butter adaptations: Butter Buds are great for butter flavor over vegetables, on baked potatoes, and in sauces. However, they don't act as a moistener, crisper, or browner. You can't substitute Butter Buds for butter in baked goods, but you can substitute nonfat yogurt (I prefer nonfat vanilla yogurt to plain yogurt because it's less tart), puréed fruits, or applesauce if the recipe calls for baking in a contained pan. To disguise the taste of applesauce, add cinnamon or pumpkin pie spice. I like to add more ripe bananas to the bananas already called for in banana bread instead of the fat ingredient.

Nuts: Any time you see nuts, use half of the amount or leave them out entirely.

Baking: In baking, instead of chocolate squares, use cocoa powder and a fat substitute like nonfat yogurt.

Dressings: Instead of using oil or mayonnaise in salad dressings, thicken with Dijon mustard or puréed vegetables like onions. Use nonfat sour cream or nonfat mayonnaise, low-fat buttermilk, puréed ricotta or cottage cheese, or nonfat milk with your vinegars.

Marinades: For marinades that typically call for an acid and an oil, dilute the acid with water, wine, fruit juice, or soy sauce instead.

Cheese: Whenever you see cheese in a recipe, use nonfat cheese or nonfat sour cream.

Rice mixes: Most rice mixes call for fat, but you can just leave it out. You won't miss it.

Bacon: For recipes that call for bacon, try adding a few drops of liquid smoke for the flavor without the fat.

Have Fun

Remember, recipes are written by people just like you, and they should be re-created according to your own individual tastes. So if the recipe calls for something you don't like, leave it out or substitute something you do like. If you are missing an ingredient, try something new. Use recipes as inspiration and guidelines, not as rules and regulations.

Baking is the exception. You can't make things rise without yeast, baking powder, or baking soda, and measuring carefully does often make a difference.

Nonfat Products

There is a vast selection of nonfat products on the market, and the flavors and qualities vary greatly. If you hate the first one you try, keep trying different brands, and you'll probably find one you like.

Become a label reader before you buy. Look at the fat grams and note the serving size—if the serving on the label is one cracker and you eat seven, keep that in mind. Also, check the list of ingredients to see if there is any added fat or if the fat comes from a whole grain in the product. Sometimes fat is added, but because of the amount of fat in the serving size, the product can legally be labeled as zero fat per serving.

There are some great national brands making fat-free cookies, desserts, and other products. But just because they are labeled "fat free" doesn't mean you can eat larger portions more often. They will probably still be high in calories, because they are full of sugar.

There are also many products out there that have been around for years and have always been fat free. Jell-O pudding is made with skim milk. Fudgesicles are a skim milk product. Cracker Jacks have always been fat free, as long as you don't eat the peanuts. Corn tortillas don't have fat. Ladyfinger cookies and angel food cake are fat free. So are Frosted Flakes and Rice Krispies marshmallow treats. Most of this stuff isn't good for you, of course, but if you are going to have a treat, you might as well choose one that is fat free.

Now to name some names. Frito-Lay baked, fat-free, and reduced fat products are great. I prefer Naturally Yours fat-free sour cream. Lifetime and Kraft fat-free cheeses are excellent. I'm not big on many of the salad dressings on the market, however. You can make your own so much better.

Keebler Elfin Delights chocolate cookies and Archway lemon drops are great. And I can't tell the difference between Campbell's Healthy Request soups and the regular higher fat, higher sodium versions.

There are plenty of fat-free microwave popcorns on the market, but I like a little fat in mine for flavor. Just use one teaspoon of oil and make it on top of the stove in a pan with a lid on it. You'll only be getting four to five grams of fat and lots of taste. Any seasonings you add to your popcorn after it's cooked will stick better if it's prepared this way.

Buy your Butter Buds in packages, not in the shaker can. They'll be easier to use in recipes like mashed potatoes, and you get a huge price break.

I've said this before, but it's worth noting here again—I don't like cooking sprays. They taste funny, they gum up your pans, and they're deceptive. Every second you spray, you are adding a gram of fat. Instead, wipe regular oil on your pan with a paper towel. As long as oil isn't moving around in your pan, you're only adding about one gram of fat.

A Few Words on Calories

I am not a calorie counter, and I don't think you should be either. However, it doesn't hurt to have a general awareness of how many calories are in certain foods. Following is a general guideline.

Protein
- *Beef*—serving size, 3.5 ounces, about the size of a deck of cards: 190 calories

- *Chicken*—serving size, 3.5 ounces or one skinless breast trimmed of fat: 150 calories

- *Pork tenderloin*—serving size, 3.5 ounces, another deck of cards: 170 calories

Fruit
- *Apple*—80 calories for a medium-sized one

- *Carrot*—30 calories for a whole one

- *Banana*—105 calories for one medium-sized—see why I don't tout these?

- *Blueberries*—82 calories for 1 cup

- *Blackberries*—80 calories for 1 cup

- *Strawberries*—45 calories for 1 cup

- *Raspberries*—61 calories for 1 cup

Fibrous vegetables

■ *Broccoli*—12 calories for ½ cup raw (23 calories for ½ cup cooked)

■ *Salad, lettuce*—5 calories for ½ cup

■ *Spinach*—6 calories for ½ cup raw (25 calories for ½ cup cooked)

■ *Green beans*—22 calories for ½ cup

Carbs

Peas, corn, winter squash, potatoes, and dried beans are really starchy carbs, not fibrous vegetables, which is reflected in the calorie counts. Compare the following:

■ *Rice*—232 calories for 1 cup brown, 223 calories for 1 cup white

■ *Beans: kidney, pinto, red, lima, navy, butter, black*—100 calories for ½ cup

■ *Black-eyed peas*—100 calories for ½ cup

■ *Green peas*—67 calories for ½ cup

■ *Potatoes*—220 calories for a medium (not a giant baker); medium is about the size of a Granny Smith apple

■ *Winter squash*—40 calories for ½ cup baked

■ *Pasta*—400 calories for 4 ounces. Read the label. If pasta comes in a bag it is usually wheat. If it comes in a box, it is often an egg noodle pasta and will be higher in fat and calories.

Dairy

■ *Nonfat milk*—86 calories for 1 cup

■ *Nonfat sour cream*—20 calories for 2 tablespoons

■ *Nonfat cottage cheese*—90 calories for ½ cup

■ *Parmesan cheese*—23 calories for 1 tablespoon grated

COOKING IN QUANTITY

The best way to live lean and eat right for a lifetime is to cook the majority of your meals at home. That's the only way you will really know how much fat you are getting. Unless you have someone to cook for you or you don't mind cooking every day, the best system is to prepare food in quantity. You can assemble a week's worth or a month's worth in just part of one day off, but you have to be efficient.

Here's how:

1. Make a list of recipes you like, then spend some time organizing them in a loose-leaf binder with plastic sheet protectors available at office supply stores. This is critical to making up your grocery list. If you get organized and stay that way, it will save you lots of time later.

2. If you can get a friend or family member to help make this more of a social experience and less of a chore, the process will go more quickly. Even if your "assistant" doesn't know how to cook and is only cleaning up for you or talking to you, it will help.

3. Plan your menu. Pick a variety of dishes. Don't make everything with potatoes. The first time you try this, choose recipes for just three meals. Pull out the recipes and make your grocery list. (Work your way up to making five meals with four portions of each.) This will take you four to six hours of cooking time and an hour of grocery shopping time, but provide you with a meal for every weeknight for a month. Choose an off-hour at your grocery to save time in line. If you are cooking for more than one person or more than one week, make sure you multiply the quantities of each ingredient.

4. Before you start cooking, figure out how many containers you need and get them ready. It would be disastrous to cook twenty meals and have nothing to put them in. Also make sure you have room in your freezer.

5. Number your meals, and as you write down the ingredients on your shopping list, note the meal number and

what you have to do to prepare it (such as chop or grate). This, too, will save you time later, especially if you have help in the kitchen and can give someone a job of chopping the onions or grating the cheese.

It's helpful to start with a clean kitchen and an empty dishwasher. And use your timers. It really takes a lot of the thought out of the process and you'll have fewer problems.

The First Steps

Now let's get started. Set out your containers, put on your apron, and turn on your TV. Your goal is never to have an empty burner.

If you have items like rice or potatoes that need to boil, put them on to cook and then begin to prep your other ingredients. It's easiest to prep the things common to several recipes first, such as garlic, onions, or peppers. For dishes like lasagne, for which you are cooking a sauce before combining ingredients and baking, start the sauce now, so you won't have to wait for it later.

Next trim all your meats.

Store food as you go. When your rice or potatoes finish, divide them into containers and let them begin to cool. If you are cooking several different kinds of chicken breast, make separate foil-divided sections on your cookie sheet, so you can put one flavor in each section and the flavors won't merge.

If something must bake or simmer for a long time, you can prepare it last and clean up the kitchen while you wait for it to cook.

If you are going to reuse things like bowls or utensils, just rinse them. Don't bother with soap and water at this point, unless they have been in contact with raw meat.

If you are cooking chicken to be frozen and the meal will be reheated, cook it just until it has changed from pink to white—20 minutes at 350 degrees is long enough and will prevent chicken from turning to leather when you reheat. Undercook pasta to al dente so you won't be eating mush.

Rely on convenience products to make things go faster— salad in bags, chopped garlic in a jar (as long as it's not stored in oil), barbecue sauce, spice mixtures, chopped cheese, and shredded cheese, carrots, or cabbage.

Use your food processor to chop large amounts of garlic (if you prefer the taste of fresh garlic) or onions or other vegetables if they are going to be cooked down to a mush. If you need some texture, you'll have to chop the old-fashioned way.

Wash and rinse everything as you go. At the end, stack similar items to be washed together, and washing will go more quickly.

Weird Cooking Tips

Things like black pepper (or any hot peppers) and garlic intensify after freezing; leafy herbs diminish in flavor. Compensate now or when you reheat. If you are winging it and cooking without a recipe, 350 degrees is the universal oven temperature for cooking anything. You won't go too far wrong. If you are cooking on top of the stove, try medium-high for everything except cheeses, which always need to be on low. Whenever you are cooking with water, always use cold water unless the recipe specifies hot water. Once you bring rice to a boil, cover it, reduce heat to simmer, turn on the timer, and leave it alone. Do not stir it unless you want it to be sticky and gummy for sushi or you plan on eating with chopsticks.

Store your food as individual meals, basically making your own TV dinners. Make sure you label all your meals: When they've been in the freezer for a month, you won't recognize them. Defrost your meals overnight in the refrigerator. Before you microwave, pop the lid and remove the label. Then reheat them on high for three minutes. You may need to alter these cooking instructions slightly according to your microwave.

C h a p t e r   S i x

NO PAIN IS GAIN: THE ANTI-AEROBICS WORKOUT

In July 1996, the U.S. Surgeon General issued a report that was as significant as its warning thirty years ago that tobacco use caused cancer. According to its research, Americans are fatter and less active than at any time in our country's history, and that very lack of exercise is directly linked to higher rates of disease and death.

The report should have sent shock waves through America.

Sadly, I don't think it did. We've all known for a long time what exercise can do for our health. But what no one has been able to answer is why so few of us are out there doing some sort of workout. Why, if a good weight workout is the one great trump card that you can play to boost health and reshape your body, have only 10 percent of American adults joined a gym? Why do so few of us even attempt the most undemanding of exercises, such as walking?

Something is seriously wrong. And I'm afraid I know exactly what it is.

Most of you don't exercise because somewhere in your unconscious mind, you think a workout has to be punishing to be successful. Remember the way you got taunted in seventh grade phys ed class when you couldn't climb the rope? Remember the humiliation of not passing the President's Council on Physical Fitness Test? I never once won that award, and it bothered me my entire youth. I felt like a loser. I didn't throw the softball well, I was too slow at the shuttle run, I was terrible at the arm hang, and I was too overweight to place in the top ten in the 12-minute run.

Although I always considered this award one for fitness, I didn't learn until years later that the activities in the test really had nothing at all to do with fitness. No one ever told me what true fitness was. Just like you, I bought into the idea that being fit means being a good athlete. I thought only the most strenuous two-hour workout could have an impact on my body. If I was not sweating profusely or having trouble breathing while working out, I thought I was doing something wrong.

Do you still accept the idea that you can only lose weight through exercise if you push your body to the limits of endurance? Do you believe all those phrases that became popular during the aerobics craze of the 1980s? "Go for the burn." "Let's get pumped!" And, of course, "No pain, no gain."

I hate the word *aerobics*. It's not that I hate what aerobics means. I hate what aerobics has come to stand for. But I've got tremendous news for you, and it's not just to make you feel good. The top researchers in the field of fitness have been saying the same thing for the last several years: We don't burn extra amounts of fat or gain extra muscle just because our lungs are gasping for oxygen and our legs are wobbly from jumping up and down.

Indeed, being in shape doesn't have anything at all to do

with being a good performer in an aerobics class or showing your stuff on a basketball court. If you can do that, that's great, and more power to you. But if your goal is to get healthy and reduce body fat, what you need to know is that developing and toning your muscles is the best, most effective kind of exercise you can do.

Moreover, when it comes to weight training, the amount of weight you lift is far less important to developing the perfect body than is the form you follow while training. Muscle soreness is not a sign of progress in shaping your hips and thighs and biceps. Good technique is.

Repeat after me. No pain is gain. Less is more. The big lie in physical fitness has been the idea that you have to grunt to get fit, that you have to pant to get lean. With the North Program, you're never going to leave the gym or a workout room feeling exhausted. Instead, you'll feel invigorated. Believe me, I walk my walk. In my own fitness clubs, I enforce a rule for 200 personal trainers I've hired. If they make any of their clients sore in the first two weeks, they'll be asked to leave.

In this chapter, I want you to forget everything you've ever heard about fitness. It's time to start all over. I know you may be anxious about this section of the book. It's been sort of fun in the earlier chapters talking about how to eat, because we all like to eat. But just the idea of putting on shorts, T-shirts, and tennis shoes and heading to a gym may fill you with dread.

I want you to know I understand that. But I want to emphasize that the dread you feel is based only on misinformation and mistaken perceptions of what exercise for fitness should be. What I want you to do in this chapter is relax.

THE TWO-PRONGED PROGRAM

There are two basic forms of exercise, both of them widely misunderstood. You need to do (1) cardiovascular exercise, which includes everything from walking, running, and aerobics classes to bicycling and swimming, and (2) weight training. Remember, one does not substitute for the other. You cannot, for example, hope to put on muscle and shape your body by doing only cardio exercise. (Have you ever noticed how long-distance runners rarely have well-developed bodies?) Nor can you hope to lose all your fat just by building your muscle through weight training. (How many overbloated guys do you see lifting weights for hours?)

If you're starting out, I recommend a cardio program that involves some sort of body movement three times a week, for at least twenty minutes each time. Weight training should be done two to three times a week for about thirty to forty-five minutes a session. That's it. If you try to do more, you won't gain anything for your efforts.

I once had a very attractive forty-year-old client named Terri who looked pretty good when she first walked into the gym, but only because she had recently been dieting herself to thinness. I asked her how she was feeling, and she told me there were days she was so listless from a lack of energy that she couldn't move. I asked her if she liked her body. She said she couldn't stand her body. "Larry, all I do is diet. There might be weeks when I'm really thin and I look good in a dress, but my body has no shape, and I have no energy. I guess all I can say is that I'm just occasionally thin, and it hasn't made me any happier."

When I asked her about working out, Terri was like so many others—completely baffled and misled by fitness myths. She told me that during those times when she walked on the treadmill, she put on extra-heavy clothes because she thought sweating meant she was losing more weight. "A complete myth," I told her. She said she never ate before a workout because she thought if her stomach was empty, her body would start to work on her excess fat during her workout. "Another myth," I said. She told me she thought that the longer she went without eating after exercise, the more fat was burned off. "Myth," I replied. And then she told me she didn't like to exercise on some days when she had a lot to do, because she believed that exercise is supposed to deprive you of energy.

"The biggest myth of all!" I bellowed.

I got Terri to start following my eating program; then I put her on the treadmill three to four times a week for 45 minutes and got her doing very light weight training three times a week. After three months—three months!—her body was transformed. She had the sleekest shoulders and arms of just about any woman I had ever seen. After thinking she was destined to spend the rest of her life being a thin, shapeless woman addicted to her diet, she told me recently, "Larry, for the first time in my entire life, I've learned to love my body."

I've learned to love my body. Those are my six favorite words in life. My goal is for you to say the very same thing.

YOUR CARDIO WORKOUT

For Terri, the key to a better body was learning how to exercise smarter, not harder. If you do a cardio exercise for a certain amount of time, your body starts to run out of its available supply of glucose and begins looking for an alternative fuel supply. So far, so good. All you have to do is get your body, when it's in that state, to burn its own fat cells for fuel.

Unfortunately, it's easier said than done. If you push yourself too hard, you can send your body into oxygen debt when you start panting. Your aerobic exercise then becomes anaerobic exercise, and your body stops burning fat because the oxygen debt builds up something called lactic acid. This acid inhibits the release of fatty acids that could otherwise be burned as fuel. Thus, if you think very intense exercise at a peak level burns pure fat, you're dead wrong. Sure, you'll burn a little fat. But to burn the most fat, scientific research says that you should only do one thing—moderate exercise of long, steady duration.

"Wait, Larry," you're probably saying, "that can't be true. If I work out at a strenuous level, surely I'm burning calories faster than if I take a walk around the park."

That's true. But here's the problem. The calories you are burning at that level are mostly coming from your valuable muscle cells. Researchers at Georgia University recently had overweight students and staff do treadmill work four times a week, expending

300 calories per session. One half did the treadmill work at high intensity while the other half went more slowly, but for a longer period, to reach the 300-calorie level. Astonishingly, both groups lost an identical amount of fat—five pounds! The point of the study? Why work harder if you don't have to?

In essence, if you want to focus on stripping fat from your body, you should slow down. Almost every day at one of my Larry North Total Fitness centers, one of my 200 personal trainers is telling a client, "Longer! Slower! Steadier!"

Now, let me be clear. If you are already very lean, you probably do need to increase slightly the intensity of your cardio exercises to get leaner. But if you have higher than average body fat, then longer and less intense cardio workouts are more important for you, to enable you to burn fat. In fact, other research has shown that when people with high body fat content increase their workout intensity, their fat burning rates remain the same. If you have a large amount of body fat, this news should make you jump for joy, because it means you don't have to kill yourself while working out.

And you should jump even higher when you take into account the fact that a moderate cardio exercise provides an array of other benefits. It strengthens your heart, improves your blood circulation, lowers your blood pressure, decreases your cholesterol, and gets rid of loads of psychological stress, making you feel better about your life.

But What is Moderate?

So what is a good cardiovascular workout, if it's not an all-out sweat-a-thon? Here's my definition: During the entire time you do a cardio exercise, you should be able to carry on a conversation. To see of you're maintaining the right level of cardio exercise, make sure you can talk to someone at any point during the exercise. You'll work up a mild sweat, which is fine. But if you can't keep a conversation going, then you're working too hard. (For most people, that would be between the 3.0 and 4.0 levels on a treadmill.)

I use this test myself. I like to be able to read when I'm on a stationary bicycle, daydream when I'm taking a brisk walk, talk to my friends when I'm on the treadmill. The goal of my cardio program is not to exhaust, but to invigorate.

So What Do I Do?

I work out at a variety of activities—outdoor walking, riding a stationary bike, and fast walking on the treadmill. My favorite outdoor activities are mountain hiking or beach walking. I do not do aerobics classes for one simple reason—I'm too uncoordinated! But it hasn't hurt me a bit. Remember, just because you're not athletic shouldn't keep you from obtaining desirable fitness goals. The best exercise is the one you enjoy the most.

I'm not going to insult your intelligence by going into long descriptions of how to jog, walk on the treadmill, or use a stationary bicycle. If you experiment with the machines at the gym, you'll find the one that suits you. Don't feel bad or inadequate because someone else is using a different machine. You're still deriving great benefits from whatever cardio exercise you have chosen. If your muscles get fatigued—or if your lungs are strained—within 30 minutes, then you're working too hard. Slow down.

Another thing to remember is that you don't need special clothes, special shoes, or a special piece of equipment to get a good cardio workout. You need thirty minutes. And really, if you want to cut down to the bare bones, just walk. Research suggests that an hour of walking at five miles per hour, done with strong arm-swinging, burns 530 calories, while an hour of light running burns just 480. (If you don't want to swing your arms, don't worry about it. You're still getting a great workout.)

And here's another piece of good news. If you are out of shape and can't go thirty minutes straight during your cardio workout, then break it up. Do fifteen minutes, ten minutes, even three minutes if you have to. Do some of it in the morning and some in the evening—any way you like—as long as you get it in. Just watch: You will build your endurance. And your fat will begin to burn.

Warming Up

Many of you feel the need to do a lot of toe-touching, leg-stretching, and trunk-twisting before you exercise. You are wasting your time. You want to stretch at the *end* of a workout instead, when your muscles are warm. (In Chapter Ten I'll give you a series of simple stretching routines that will give you the flexibility you need.) If you stretch your muscles when they are cold, you could tear muscle fibers, causing injury. I recommend that you start with a few minutes of easy walking or cycling on a stationary bike. This kind of warm-up is a great way to prevent injury and punch up your cardiovascular system. Don't ever try to shock your body into getting fit. You'll only be setting yourself up for pain.

Burning Fat without Working Out

It may surprise you to know that your cardio workout, no matter how long it is, is not the most significant activity you'll do to burn fat during a day. Ninety percent of the fat you burn each day is burned just doing whatever it is you do—a lot of which is just sitting down. One of the problems about living in the late twentieth century is that you can get so many things done in life with the push of a button. Two generations ago, people used a scythe to cut the grass. A generation ago, they used a push mower. Today, they use a riding lawnmower or hire someone else to cut the grass.

The U.S. Surgeon General's Report says your health is vastly improved simply by moving around more. Have you heard the old saying, "Sitting is better than lying, standing is better than sitting?" Well, it's true. According to one study, between sitting quietly and standing quietly, there's a difference of about nine calories burned an hour.

So I want you to take that extra step—literally. At the moment, it won't seem like much. But over a year's time, you will have burned off an amazing number of extra calories doing what I like to call mini cardio workouts—that is, doing a little extra when you clean your house, garden, or shop, or wash and wax your car. Here are some tips:

1. Consciously lengthen your stride every time you walk somewhere. The effect will be to increase your energy output naturally.

2. Where there are elevators or escalators, there have to be stairs. Climbing burns twice as many calories as walking on a level floor. So why ride one or two floors when you can walk them?

3. Choose the nondriving opportunity. Walk or ride a bicycle instead of driving to a nearby location. Park your car in the most distant space in a parking lot instead of looking for a spot near the door.

4. Find ways to move around in your office. Walk to the more distant water cooler rather than the one by your desk. Walk to the corner mailbox. Pace around your office when you're thinking. At the least, don't sit for more than an hour without getting up and stretching for a few minutes.

5. Don't hesitate to participate in light recreational sports—shooting baskets, playing kickball or Ping-Pong with the kids, joining in a pickup volleyball game. Somewhere inside you, fat will be burned.

6. When you feel like napping, take a walk instead. You'll discover you are more refreshed. Exercise has a better psychological effect than napping. It causes the release of endorphins that give you a kind of light euphoria. Endorphins have been described as emotional tranquilizers that reduce anxiety. They're the best natural response to stress that our bodies produce.

Tips For Effective Cardio Workouts

1. It's a good idea to cross-train—to vary your cardio choices. Walk one day, cycle the next, and take a swim on the third. Cross-training develops a more balanced state of fitness. It also helps reduce the risk of injury. If you find one you like, it's okay to stick with it.

2. Drink plenty of water before and after exercise. It is an old wives' tale that lack of water during a workout helps you lose weight. It is also a myth that you'll get stomach

cramps if you drink water during a workout. Water is the essence of life. The weight of a typical male body is made up of 60 percent water, that of a female, 50 percent. Part of the problem we encounter when exercising is that our water loss easily exceeds our ability to replace it. And when dehydration exceeds 2 percent of our body weight, physical performance is impaired. Additionally, when you feel a need to drink water because you're thirsty, it is already too late: You're already dehydrated. So it's very important that you maintain your fluid intake at all times. For every pound you lose from cardio exercise, you should drink one pint of water. Only old-fashioned football coaches think you get in better shape by dehydrating yourself while exercising.

3. As for the question of when to exercise, I'm not one to say you have to work out exactly at the same time every day; however, your body thrives on regularity and consistency. If you work out early in the morning, several things will happen. First, you'll find that you want to eat healthfully throughout the day, because you have worked out and feel so good about yourself that you won't want to blow it on a bad meal. Second, a morning workout means you don't have to worry about what may happen at the end of the day, when you might have to pick up the kids or be on time for a dinner engagement. If you can't fit in a morning workout, what about lunchtime? You don't need an hour to eat. You can eat one of the meals I've described in Chapter Three in ten minutes. After you've eaten, why don't you put on a pair of tennis shoes and walk for thirty minutes? In your car, keep gym bag filled with workout gear. You'll be amazed at the opportunities you'll find to work out.

What Not to Expect from Cardio

There's going to come a moment when you're on a StairMaster or treadmill at the gym and some hard-bodied type is going to get on a machine beside you and go at full speed. When that happens, you're inevitably going to think that you should be doing the same thing. You'll think, "Maybe Larry's right about me getting leaner through slower exercise. But if I want a true hard body, then I need more cardio."

Sorry, but a longer, harder cardio workout is not a shortcut to a harder body. Additional cardio exercise beyond sixty minutes will not give you results that are significantly greater than what you'll get from 60 minutes. Think about it. If all it took to get a lean beautiful body was doing cardio exercise an hour a day, six days a week, then everyone would have a lean body.

The truth is that a lean body requires a total, multifaceted program—cardio, eating, and weight training. You can't depend on a long cardio workout to get rid of that extra piece of cake you ate the night before, and you can't depend on a cardio workout to permanently speed up your metabolism. Don't forget, what speeds up your metabolism is more muscle tissue, which means a program of weight training. Excessive cardio exercise can actually hurt your muscle development. If you do too much cardio, your body will pull nutrients from your muscles. Such exercise reduces fat. It does not shape your body.

Weight training! If you're tempted to close the book right now, thinking to yourself that there's no way you're going to start lifting weights, stop right there. Turn the page and just read. When you finish Chapter Seven, you'll be ecstatic about the potential you have to transform your body.

THE FOUNTAIN OF YOUTH: DEVELOPING THE BEST BODY OF YOUR LIFE

I know, I'm repeating myself. Muscle is the most valuable commodity in your body. Muscle is to your body what gold is to the economy. It's your fountain of youth.

Think of the more than 400 muscles in your body that keep it firm or allow it to sag. Each muscle is composed of millions of tiny cells. There's no other way around it: To make those cells work, you've got to use them. Allowing a muscle to go unused not only

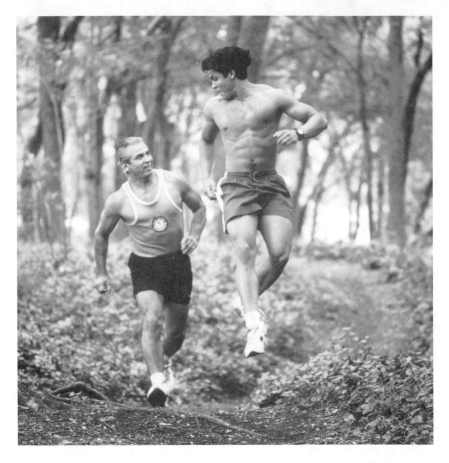

compromises your health, but it also keeps you from full physical potential. Not as much blood travels through an unused muscle, which means that muscle won't get enough oxygen and calcium, and that means your tendons and ligaments become fragile. Eighty percent of all lower back pain may be attributed to muscular deficiency rather that pathology. Often, all you need to lick your back problems is a stronger back and legs. And the only way to get a stronger back is weight training.

And if you're a woman, listen to this: Studies show that you are more likely to develop osteoporosis—a condition in which your bones weaken and you start to hunch over as you get older—than are men. You already have lower bone density than a man, and after menopause you lose even more. One great way to combat this loss is weight training. Your bones, which grow more brittle with age, actually gain more calcium and get stronger through weight training.

Weight training works, plain and simple. The best-shaped and most attractive bodies in the world—from Olympic athletes to basketball players to fashion models—get their forms from some form of weight training. If you give your muscles just a little resistance, your body's youthful contours will start to return. You improve your posture and carriage, your saggy skin tightens, and your lungs provide more oxygen.

Most people believe that when they hit a certain age—usually forty—their body shape will never again be the same. It's not true. Weight training is the easiest body makeover there is. It can give a man firm biceps and an upper back as wide as an eagle's wingspan. It can give a woman nice, shapely legs, a small waist, and tight hips. Just think, with simple weight training exercises, you can lose your thunder thighs and saddlebags. Your "love handles" will melt away. Believe me, it's a lot less painful and inexpensive than surgery.

Plagued by prevailing myths, you may never have seriously tried it. Maybe you think you can't put on muscle at your age, so it's pointless to start. Or maybe you're afraid that the lightest weight will make you develop masculine muscles or pump you up. Or, if you're male, you may think too much muscle will turn to fat the moment you stop working out.

Wrong, wrong, wrong. Weightlifters who look bloated and fat are not that way because of their weight training. They are that way because of bad eating habits that have not starved the fat while feeding the muscle. If you're following the eating program and doing your cardio workouts, then weight training in the most modest amounts—which is what I recommend and *all* that I recommend—is going to produce results. You'll immediately began shedding your fat layer and rejuvenating your long-dormant muscle tissue, building its elasticity and strength.

Will You Become a Musclehead?

More than one person has said that he's a little uncomfortable at the idea of working out with me, because I may be a musclehead. They think I'm the type who spits into the water fountain and shouts "Get huge!" "Do just one more!" "Yeah! Yeah!"

Here's the real story. The weight-training routines that you're about to discover are no different from those I follow myself. I'm not telling you one thing in this book while I am secretly sneaking off to get in a couple of extra workouts a day.

Remember how our parents watched Jack LaLanne? He is a hero of mine, a man I will always admire because of the way he converted millions of people to fitness. But Jack was—and still is—a workout fanatic. I'm not that way. And you don't need to be, either. You don't have to be a workout fanatic to look great.

I admit I have stolen a few pages from the bodybuilder playbook. Whether you love them or hate them, bodybuilders have attained a muscular development and body-fat level that was unheard of years ago. But I am not going to make a bodybuilder out of you. In the North Program, you are never going to "get huge." You are not going to build gigantic, bulging muscles. Nor will you ever have to get sore. Instead of trying to lift as much as you can, you'll develop movements with weights that are deliberate and controlled, focusing on the muscles you're supposed to be working.

Remember, in my program, more weight is not great. To me, pain only means one thing—you're hurting. No pain is gain!

HOME OR GYM?

Should you work out at home or in a gym? The advantages of having a home gym are mostly related to convenience. It's open twenty-four hours a day, for one thing, and you save a lot of exercise time if you don't have to travel to a gym. Beyond convenience, you have complete privacy.

After watching thousands of people walk into one of my gyms, I know what feelings of discomfort you may have about gym life. Compared to those who've been working out there for years, you may feel more out of shape than you really are, and that everyone is staring right at you. You may react one of two ways: (1) Back up like a crab and disappear forever out the front door, or (2) Work out so hard, trying to impress or keep up with everyone around you, that you overdo and end up so sore the next day that you can't even get out of bed.

But the fact is that people in a gym are much more concerned about themselves and aren't really paying attention to you. Moreover, the advantage of a gym (which can be a private health club, a recreational center, or even a high school weight room) is that you get better equipment and constant supervision from trainers. You can also find a workout partner who can help you tremendously, and you're likely to be further motivated simply by being around other motivated people. What you *don't* want to do at the gym is turn it into your social center, where you walk from machine to machine visiting with people.

Although I think you need to go to a gym as you become more advanced (because of the variety of things you can do), you can certainly get great results at home. To accommodate your workout, no matter the venue, I've made sure to include in Chapter Eight, on Weight Training, exercises that can be done at home as well as at the gym.

Working Out at Home

Can you develop a North Body at home? The answer is yes. You don't even need all that much equipment, so it shouldn't cost much money. It's very easy, in fact, to do the North Program with just a couple of dumbbells. A couple of lightweight dumbbells, which will cost from $10 to $30, will do just fine.

Unless you've got money to burn, you do not need one of those home stack units. I've yet to see a single one I like that is under $2,500; you'll likely get bored or grow out of them quickly, so they're not a great investment. For the initial North Body weight program, you can put together a great home gym for no more than $200. If you look in the classified ad sections of the newspapers, you'll always find used weights for sale. (These are usually from people who worked out a couple times and then gave it up. Obviously, they are not people who've read this book!)

Eventually, you may want to buy a bench that lies flat but can adjust to forty-five-degree and ninety-degree angles. At that point I'd recommend an upgrade to fixed dumbbells. They're worth their weight in gold, and you'll never have to replace them. They cost about thirty to forty cents a pound. Skip plastic weights or weights that screw off and on. You want something that feels solid in your hand. You'll also need a straight bar with various barbell plates to add to it.

If you're female, start with the following:

1. A variety of dumbbells between three and fifteen pounds.

2. A straight bar with two two-and-a-half pound plates, two five-pound plates, and four ten-pound weights.

3. With a bench, the total cost should be less than $100, hundreds less than you could probably pay for some infomercial equipment.

If you're male, start with the following:

1. Dumbbells ranging from ten to forty pounds.

2. A straight bar with four five-pound plates, four ten-pound plates, two twenty-five pound plates, and if you want, two thirty-five or forty-five pound plates.

3. With a bench, the total should be less than $250.

You can probably get the recommended equipment even cheaper if you shop around. Try to go to the gym before starting a home program, just to get a chance to see which weights will be most comfortable for you. Absolutely do not start a program without getting at least a couple of supervised sessions at a gym from an experienced weight trainer who can guide you and show you how to do the exercises properly.

And even if you have the best home gym possible, go to a public gym once every couple of months to try out its equipment and see what exercises produce the results you want. As you get more advanced, you'll probably graduate from your home operation to a commercial gym.

Working Out at the Gym

What kind of gym should you look for? First, it should be a serious, well-equipped gym where people go to train, not to socialize. I also suggest finding a gym close to your work or home, so you won't feel inconvenienced by the notion of a workout. Location, you'll learn, is one of the main determining factors of your workout. If you can't afford $20 to $150 a month for a private club,

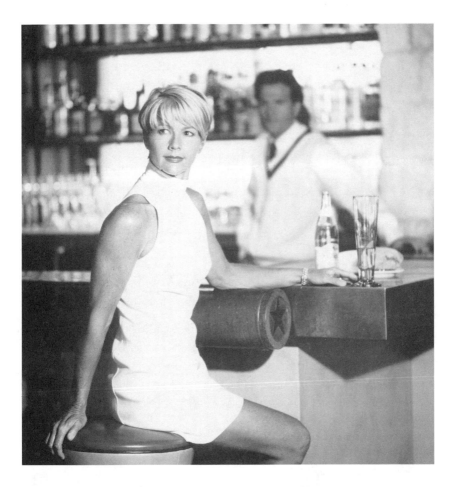

try the local high school, community college, or recreation center.

After a speech I gave in a small town, a few women came up to me and said, "Larry, our problem is that we don't have a gym to go to in this town." I asked, "Do you have a high school?" They said yes, but it was full of students. "Well," I said, "go ask the coach about using it on weekends or nights." A few weeks later, I got a letter from one of the women, who informed me that fifteen of them were meeting at the high school gym three times a week.

Some gyms are certainly expensive, but they usually have different membership rates throughout the year. The off-season in the gym world is late summer; you can get discounts of up to 50 percent if you join then. But before you join, ask yourself if you really need an expensive gym; whether you'll really take advantage of the juice bars, saunas, or massage rooms.

When picking a gym, be alert for these things:

1. If the salesman at the gym is treating you like a witness on the stand, forcing you to give testimony about your body, walk out. He may try to make you feel so bad about being out of shape that you'll pay a lot of money to join. Don't take any high-pressure tactics.

2. Study the contract closely, looking for any hidden fees.

3. Visit the club at the time of day you plan to use it. It is one thing to like a club when you're there on a lunch break, but if you're going to use it at 6:00 P.M., you need to see how crowded it is at that time.

4. Take your time looking the gym over. If the salesperson is rushing you, you need to wonder if something is wrong.

5. If you're going to change clothes at the gym, spend time in the locker room. If you're going to feel uncomfortable or unclean taking a shower and dressing there, look for another club. You'd be amazed how little things such as discomfort can keep you out of your own gym.

Do I Need a Trainer?

This book is designed to be your trainer. If you want to get a personal trainer, that's great, but expect to pay from $35 to $125 an hour. Make sure your trainer will not only supervise a weight program for you but also can understand the nutrition and eating plan found in this book.

The great advantage of a trainer is that he or she can keep you motivated. If your trainer doesn't make you feel determined to do your workout, then move on to another one.

Even with a personal trainer, however, this book will serve as a reference for workouts to do long after you stop using a trainer. Your first three to six weight sessions with a trainer should be considered mostly instructional lessons, not pure workouts. Don't expect the first couple of workouts to produce significant results in your physique, but know that the next 120 workouts certainly will. One big mistake people make is that they go into their first weight training expecting to train really hard. Relax. You're there initially to learn.

REPS AND SETS

This may sound really elementary, but just so we all know we're on the same page here, I'll explain that to complete a weight-training exercise properly, you must do that exercise a certain number of times. Each time you do a single movement, it's called a *rep*—for repetition. A number of reps done together is called a *set*. If I tell you to do ten reps, then you should do the movement ten times.

Some people will tell you to rest 30 seconds between sets; others say to wait 60 seconds between sets. I suggest you rest as long as you need to. Pay attention to your body. Larger muscle groups and heavier exercises will require a little bit more rest than smaller muscle groups and lighter exercises.

Here are some guidelines for weight training sets:

1. First set: Choose a weight with which you can perform ten reps with perfect form. If you can do fifteen perfect reps, then you know you've picked a weight that's too light for you.

2. Second set: You should be able to get in eight or nine perfect reps with perfect form, but the last rep should cause a slight flaw in your form. Offsetting the weight is the challenge. Do not yank, twist, or cheat to finish the set.

3. Third set: Try again for the same effect you got in the second set. You may have to drop a little bit of weight to get in eight or nine perfect reps, or you may add a tiny iota of body torque to get the weight up for that final rep. On days where you feel weak, tired, or sore, do all three sets at the same level as your first set.

Form Is Everything

Technique determines whether you improve in weight training. The amount of weight you're moving is never the measure of your success. You must never sacrifice form for weight. I'll be repeating this mantra over and over as I take you through specific exercises. Never sacrifice form so you can finish an exercise.

The secret to good form is posture. In life, you don't have to walk around as if you're a Marine standing at attention. But you do need to be aware of posture when you lift weights. You will rarely ever see a weight movement performed incorrectly by someone who has perfect posture. Correct posture in almost every exercise means your back stays straight, your shoulders stay back, your chest sticks out, and your legs remain straight but not locked in position. If you find your shoulders slumping, your back rounding off, your hips thrusting forward, or your back jerking, then you are lifting incorrectly—and dangerously.

As you begin, the pace of your reps is very important. Slow it down. Try for rhythmic consistency. The key word to remember is *control*. You must control the weight. If you are losing control of the movement, you're doing it too fast. If you are going fast just to get the weight up, you're using too much weight. After the first several reps of an exercise, you should feel the muscle working. If you don't, you are doing your reps too quickly.

Range of Movement

In your weight-training program, you always want to get to the fullest range of motion you can. How many people do you see in a weight room doing half-movements with a lot of weight? You see them do a standard barbell curl about halfway up, then let it back down—but not all the way. If they would cut their weight in half and perform a full motion, they would get the desired results three times as quickly.

With the exception of only a couple of movements for your legs and certain back exercises (which we will talk about later), you are trying to get a full contraction when you lift the weight up and a full extension when you drop it down. If you find yourself stopping midway through the movement, you are using too much weight. Remember, with proper form, you can get as much benefit out of a light weight as you could using a heavier weight with sloppier form.

Keep Moving

You do not want to hold the weight at the top or the bottom of the movement. Keep it moving, to keep constant tension in your muscles throughout the set. And don't ever rest the bar on your chest or lock and hold it for a couple of seconds at the top—that can lead to injury. Your weight-training program should be a constant flow of motion, almost like rowing a boat without ever allowing the oars to stop moving.

Breathing

This seems silly. Everyone breathes, right? Wrong. A lot of people hold their breath when they lift, which causes them to tense up and use muscles that don't need to be involved in a particular exercise. Get in the habit of being relaxed in the weight room. That means not gripping the bar so tightly that your knuckles turn white, not grimacing or clenching your teeth. And most importantly, it means breathing naturally. The only muscle group that should be tense is the muscle that you're working at the time.

When you start, it's important to lift weights with your mouth open. As you become more advanced, you will want to exhale as you lift the weight, then inhale as you let the weight down. But for now, just breathe, Make sure to inhale at the beginning of each movement.

Focus

In weight training, you've got to concentrate as if you were driving on a crowded highway. I see too many people's minds wandering as they train. You've got so many things to think about—breathing, posture, range of motion—that you shouldn't have time to think about anything else. Learn to feel every exercise you perform. Learn to focus directly on the muscle you're supposed to be working. Often you will hear an experienced weight lifter say, "Feel the movement" or "feel the muscle." It takes time and concentration, but if you can do it, you will improve vastly. Try not to miss too many workouts. Completing your worst workout is better than not working out at all.

Try Not to Get Sore

Once again, don't be fooled into thinking muscle soreness is a sign of muscle toning. Safe and sane is the technique we are going for. Your muscles don't get tighter or bigger because they get sore. The feeling you want to strive for is a pulling sensation that stretches the muscle naturally.

Rest Your Body

Here is another one of those ironies that doesn't at first glance seem logical: Your muscles will not get any stronger if you do not let them rest.

Anyone who tries to lift weights twice a day is doomed. You should lift weights three times a week at most. After being exercised intensely, a muscle needs about forty-eight—sometimes 72—hours of rest to make its best progress. Overtraining can lead to injury, but it can also lead to muscle loss. That's right. It's possible to wear down the muscle so much it won't have the strength to grow.

Weight workouts shouldn't last longer than sixty minutes; sometimes thirty minutes is all you need. They need to be done at a good comfortable pace, and you should try to develop a nice rhythm as you progress from one movement to another. Don't feel you have to spend a long time on any particular exercise.

Now you are ready to hit the weightroom! Just as you do with your eating program, try to get into the habit of being very consistent with your workouts for the first six weeks. Although missing a couple of workouts isn't going to jeopardize your progress, you'll find that your body will thrive on a regular workout, especially at the beginning. If you're diligent about your workout schedule, your body will develop more quickly.

Also, make sure that you start a workout diary to record each exercise. Check off each routine as you finish it, and bathe in the glow of accomplishment.

Okay, let's get to it.

Chapter Eight

WEIGHT TRAINING: THE SIMPLE STEPS TO RESHAPING YOUR BODY

People are always asking me what the "ideal" exercise is for this or that body part. In search of desired results, they latch onto the latest thing they see someone else trying in the gym. I'm sorry, but there is no secret exercise. There is no ideal movement. Basically, I'm showing you the same movements that have been performed since weight-lifting began. Yes, you'll see different people doing different routines, and at some point you should consult an expert for advanced bodywork. But for now, I'll just introduce you

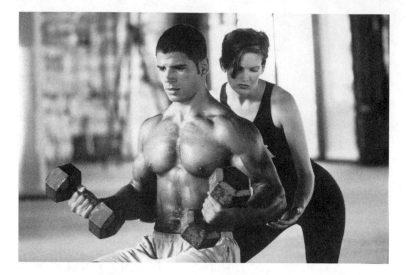

to the exercises that are the easiest to complete and have provided the best and fastest results over the years.

In this chapter, here's what you'll find:

1. For each body part, you'll first see an illustrated explanation of a simple exercise you can do at home with dumbbells or a barbell.

2. Then you'll see additional exercises for those of you who work out at a gym and have access to certain machines. You'll notice that some of these exercises also require only dumbbells or barbells, so feel free to try these at home, too, if you wish. These routines may seem simple, but again, try to stay focused on your own progress and goals, and don't worry about what you may see other people doing. Many people who train without knowledge miss out on the effectiveness of the fundamentals. That's the reason it takes so long for their bodies to graduate to intermediate or advanced levels. This program hits every muscle group and will remain your solid foundation forever.

Go Slowly

Whether you've been a gym-goer previously or you've never set foot in a gym before, do one thing for me. Go slowly. Don't try to lift very much in your first weeks. If you get sore—which you shouldn't, if you follow my instructions—then you'll end up in bed the next morning, hardly able to move and cursing me the whole time. That's not what we want, is it? So, for your sake as well as mine, ease into the program one step at a time.

1. *First week:* Perform only one exercise for each of the body parts I discuss here. That means one chest exercise, one back exercise, and so on. Do only one set of ten reps, using a weight that does not require any strain whatsoever. Worry about form only, not weight. Your first few weight workouts should last maybe fifteen to twenty minutes each. If, at the end of the first week, you feel it's too easy, then you're getting it right.

2. *Second week:* Keep doing only one exercise per body part, but move up to two sets per exercise for the major muscle groups, while remaining at a one-set level for the smaller muscle groups. Continue to avoid any strain. If you still feel it's too easy and you're thinking, "Come on, let me at these weights," then you are going at the perfect pace.

3. *Third week:* You're going to pick up the intensity gradually. Do two exercises, two sets each, on your major muscle groups. Then do one exercise, two sets each, on your minor muscle groups. Pick and choose weights with which you are comfortable and confident. Absolutely no straining! By the end of the third week, try for the regular routine that follows.

The Regular Routine

When you're ready for the regular routine, here's all you have to do:

1. Pick out two exercises for each larger muscle group category. That means two exercises for the chest, two for the back, two for the shoulders, two for the glutes, and two for

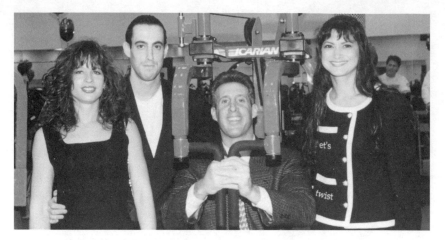

My sister-in-law Joan, brother Alan, me, and Melanie
at the opening of one of my gyms.

the quads. You'll do two or three sets of ten reps each of
each exercise.

2. Pick out one exercise for each smaller muscle group. Of
each exercise, you'll do two to three sets for biceps, triceps, hamstrings, and calves.

3. Keep each session no longer than forty to sixty minutes.
You should do your weight routines two to three times a
week for the next six to eight weeks. Nothing more. Don't
think that because two sets feel good, five sets will feel
even better. That's a classic mistake. Once you've
learned the exercises and your body has acquired some
stamina, your goal should be to do three perfect sets—
but no more. You don't want to overwork your muscles.

On those days that you feel a little fatigued, don't miss a
workout—just perform your sets at a much lighter level, so you
can get in ten reps with perfect form and not worry about straining. You'll still be amazed at how much your muscles respond.
But when you do feel your muscles respond, don't get paranoid
and think you're starting to bulk up. You are not spending the
hundreds of hours in the gym that bodybuilders do to train for
muscle size. This is training for a more balanced, defined
physique. Besides, most of the bulk you see in them is fat. Because
you are melting away fat, what you're getting is tone.

MAJOR MUSCLE GROUPS

The Chest Exercises

Let's start with the glory body part. Men see a strongly developed chest as the ultimate symbol of masculine strength. Women think of stronger pecs as their chance to get bigger breasts. Actually, chest exercises won't change the size of the mammary glands, but they will keep your breasts from sagging. By strengthening your pectoral muscles, you'll make your breasts firmer simply by giving them a muscular foundation.

At home:

Flat bench press

The flat bench press is the world's oldest weight-lifting movement, and perfect to work all of your chest muscles.

1. Using dumbbells or a barbell, lie down on a flat bench. Grab the bar a little wider than shoulder width.

2. Now push straight up so the weights are directly above your chest (or even directly above your eyes).

3. Slowly bring the weight back down to the top part of your chest.

Tips:

- You want your elbows pointed outward, but do not force them too far back, because that will put unnecessary stress on your shoulders.

- Keep your feet firmly planted on the floor at all times, and do not lock your arms at the top of the movement.

At the gym:

Incline press

The incline press is not as stressful on your back and will help develop the usually neglected upper chest better than the traditional flat bench press. Keep in mind that in the traditional bench press, men tend to use too much weight and end up straining too hard.

The incline press can be done with either barbells or dumbbells. *Note to women:* If using a barbell, you should start with fifteen to twenty pounds total weight. Since a regular-sized barbell weighs that much, you don't need to add extra weight. If you're using dumbbells, start with eight pounds in each hand. *Note to men:* Start with forty-five to sixty-five pounds total weight on a barbell, or fifteen- to twenty-pound dumbbells.

1. Using either a barbell or dumbbells, lie with your back flat on a 45-degree-angle bench. Elbows should stick out parallel from your shoulders.

2. Push up and back, almost in an arc over your head. Most people make a mistake in pushing too far out in front of them. If you go out instead of straight up, you'll work more of your shoulders than your chest. It's important to stretch fully at the bottom of the movement and to flex the chest as you push up.

Tips:

- If you use dumbbells, push up with your palms forward, and be sure to push in a triangular motion, so that the dumbbells come up like a pyramid. At the top, the dumbbells should come close together but never touch.

- Obviously, these are easy to do at home if you have an inclined bench.

Flat bench flies

This is not like a "press," in which you take the weights up and down. Here, in order to enhance the cleavage of your pecs, you move the arms as if you're flying.

1. With a dumbbell in each hand, extend your arms fully above you while lying on a flat bench. As you go down, keep the arms straight but not locked; keep a slight bend in the elbows. You want to bring the weight down only until your arms are parallel to the ground.

2. Move your arms back up, bringing the weights to a point about three to five inches from each other. Pretend you have a barrel on your chest and that you are trying to bring the dumbbells around the outside of the barrel.

Tips:

- You want the weights to be above your chest when you're at the top of the movement and parallel with your shoulders at the bottom of the movement. *Note:* you can do this exercise on a 45-degree-angle incline bench to work your upper chest, or a decline bench to work your lower chest.

■ Avoid bending your elbows too far or locking them straight out.

The pec deck

Another great cleavage-building exercise.

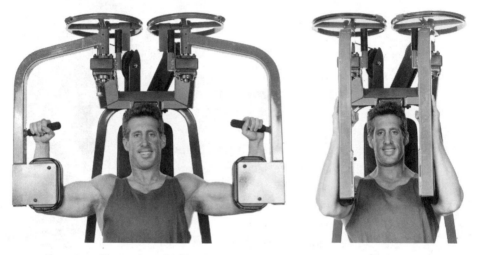

1. Sit in the chair of the machine and adjust the seat so that a straight line could be drawn between the bottom part of your elbow and the lower part of your shoulder.

2. Let the weight stretch your arms back so you can feel a stretch across your chest.

3. Slowly bring the weight all the way forward, squeezing and flexing the chest the entire time.

Tips:

■ Avoid adjusting the seat too high, making your elbows too low and your head too far forward.

■ If you have any shoulder problems, avoid this machine entirely.

Chest press machine

A great exercise for the entire chest.

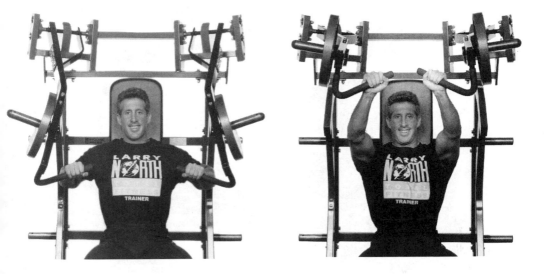

1. Adjust the seat so that your hands are just below your shoulders. Then position yourself so that your back is straight.

2. Now push forward, tensing your chest the entire time. Straighten your arms, but do not allow your shoulders to overextend.

3. Return the weight to the starting position and repeat.

Tip:

■ Don't roll your shoulders, and keep your back straight against the pad at all times.

Dips

For your lower chest.

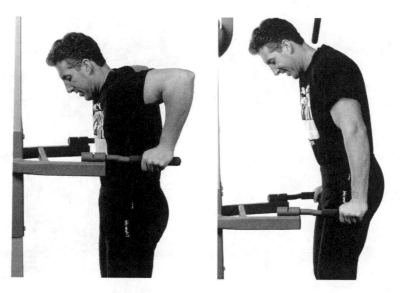

1. Put your hands on the bars beside your body.

2. Dip down deep enough to get a good stretch in the chest.

3. When you come back up, don't lock with your arms. Come up only about three-quarters of the way. Always keep focused on the chest muscle, trying to keep it tense.

Tips:

- When doing dips, you want the elbows out, not in.
- Avoid bending your back at all times.

The Back Exercises

■ The back gets neglected more than any body part, mainly because you can't see it most of the time. You have to concentrate when working on your back, because you have an array of different muscles in your upper, middle, and lower back. If you have undeveloped back muscles, your shoulder blades will stick out like big bony knobs. An undeveloped upper back will also make your waist look wide. Ideally, you want your upper body to taper into a tight V as it comes to your waist—and to do that, you've got to build your back.

In each of the following exercises, pay a lot of attention to keeping your back straight, because you'll hurt your lower back if you are working out in a bent-over position. Also, make sure not to grip the bar of your weight too tightly, as that will make the arm muscles do too much of the work. If you lighten up on your grip and practice stretching your back between sets, you'll learn to feel your back muscles doing the work.

At home:

One-arm dumbbell rows

For the muscles directly in the
middle of your back.

1. Put your left knee on a flat
   bench and keep your
   right foot on the floor.
   With the dumbbell in
   the right hand, lean over
   and put your free (left)
   hand on the front part
   of the bench to support
   yourself.

2. With the weight dropped all
   the way down, rotate your
   shoulder upward as you
   lift the dumbbell to your
   waist.

3. Slowly let the weight
   back down, feeling
   the back muscles
   stretch until your arm is
   fully extended.

4. Repeat the movement
   on the other side by switching legs and switching the
   weight to the opposite hand.

Tips:

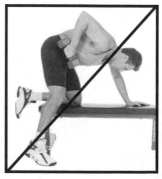

■ Don't let the weight go straight
  down. Bring the weight down at an
  angle so that it ends up at the front
  of your body.

■ Always keep your back straight.
  And never pull with your shoulders

or jerk the weight up, or you'll hurt your lower back. If you feel compelled to jerk, stop the exercise immediately and get a lighter weight.

At the gym:

Bent-over row

This is like the exercise you just learned, only it involves two arms and a barbell. It also works the middle of the back.

1. Keeping your knees slightly bent, bend over until your back is parallel with the ground. Bend your knees to pick up the bar, and keep your hands shoulder-width apart. You can use an overhand grip or underhand grip.

2. With your shoulders straight, chest out, pull the bar to the lower chest or the upper stomach. Then slowly let it back down so your arms are fully extended.

3. As you pull upward, pull the shoulders back as if you are trying to make your shoulder blades touch. It's harder to breathe in this position, which makes it important to concentrate on your breathing.

Tip:

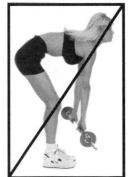

■ Avoid bending or bowing your back and shoulders. Do not raise your torso during the movement. Perform the exercise in front of a mirror, if possible, so you can tell if you're using proper form.

Lat pull-downs

For the muscles right underneath the armpits that give your back a beautiful V-shape.

1. Using either a close-together grip or a wide grip, grab the bar above you and pull it down to the top of the chest or the bottom of the chin. Pulling any lower works the shoulders more than the back.

2. Let the weight up, extending your arms until they are straight up. As you do so, allow your torso to straighten out completely.

Tips:

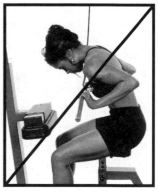

■ Don't pull the bar behind your head, as it puts undue stress on your neck and lower back.

■ The key to lat pull-downs is the extension. As you pull down, allow your back to sway back very slightly.

■ Avoid leaning back too far. Keep your shoulders back and your back straight.

Machine row

For the muscles in the middle region of the back.

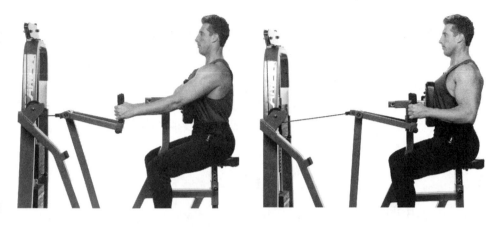

1. Sit in the machine, keeping your back perfectly straight.

2. Grab the handles, pulling with your shoulders and back, bringing the weight back.

3. Move forward with the weight fully extended, but don't allow your back to round out.

Tip:

■ Pull with a softer hand grip, so you won't be using too much of your arm strength. Don't let your hips move too far forward.

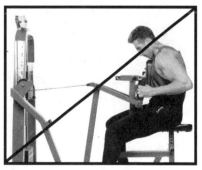

The Shoulder Exercises

■ Strong shoulders are one of the keys to good posture. They give width to the upper body, which in turn makes your waist look smaller. Since your shoulders comprise a very small muscle group and get worked in every upper-body exercise you do, these exercises don't require a lot of weight. However, the shoulders are an easy muscle group to overtrain and injure, so you should certainly work them carefully. If you have a shoulder injury or shoulder problem—which can mean any type of pain in that area—you might consider skipping these exercises.

At home:

Upright row

A great overall exercise for all the shoulder muscles.

1. With your hands six to eight inches apart as they hold the barbell (you can also use dumbbells), stand up with your back perfectly straight and your feet a little closer together than shoulder width. Keep your legs slightly bent.

2. Starting off with your arms extended straight down, pull the bar or the dumbbells to your chin. Keep the knuckles of your hands pointed down at the ground during the entire movement, and keep the bar as close to your body as possible.

3. Keep your elbows higher than the bar through the movement. Let the bar down so you can get a complete stretch at the bottom. Repeat.

Tip:

- Avoid leaning too far back. Keep your back perfectly straight, your hands at least six inches apart, and your elbows higher than the barbell.

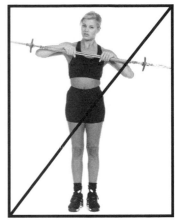

At the gym:

Side Lateral Raises

An exercise to broaden the middle muscles of the shoulders.

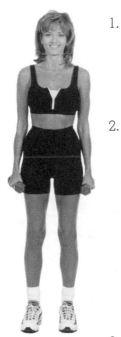

1. Women, use three-to-five pound dumbbells. Men, start with eight-to-ten pound dumbbells. Either stand or sit on a bench or chair. Gripping your dumbbells, drop your hands all the way down to your sides.

2. In a smooth and deliberate movement, send the arms and dumbbells straight out to the side at right angles from your body. Try to keep the arms straight, without locking. Your hands should always be in line with the shoulders.

3. Let the dumbbells down slowly. Think of performing this movement the way a ballet dancer does, slowly, with fluidity.

Tips:

- When you raise them, the dumbbells should barely go higher than shoulder level.

- Don't move your arms forward or jerk them. If you have to use a jerking movement, it means you're using too much weight. Your arms should move out smoothly.

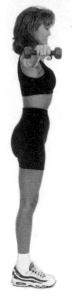

Front Lateral Raises

For the front muscles of the shoulders.

1. Start with the dumbbells in front of your body.

2. Bring them up slowly so they are a little bit higher than your shoulders.

3. Let the weight down slowly, with control, then repeat. Try to stay in motion the whole time.

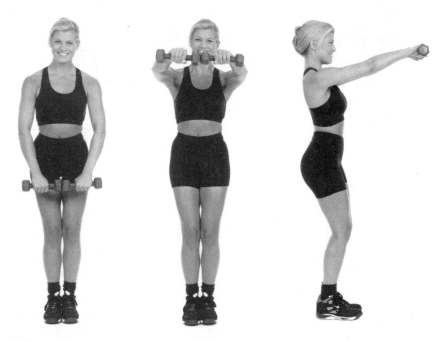

- This movement needs to be done very slowly, without swinging. Don't do it if it hurts your shoulders.

Overhead Press

For your overall shoulder muscles. Whether you're using a machine, dumbbells, or barbells, perform this exercise seated to prevent back strain.

1. Seated properly, keeping your back flush against the back pad, hold the bar (or dumbbell) at shoulder width. Push the weight straight overhead, but not behind your head.

2. Let the weight back down slowly, and repeat.

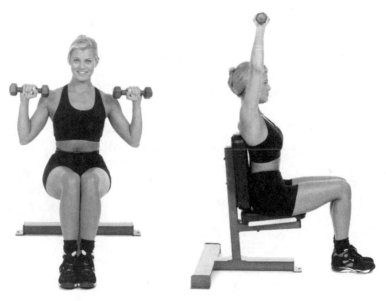

T i p :

- Avoid lifting if you are already fatigued, and never go too heavy. These are smaller muscles, and they don't require much weight. Also, don't do this movement if you have back problems.

The Leg Exercises (Glutes and Quads)

The big leg muscles are often neglected. For people training at home, there is little equipment to help them train their legs. Most men are usually so concerned with their upper bodies that they have a tendency to blow off leg workouts. Women tend to ignore leg training for fear they will develop overly large muscles in their legs.

Despite all these issues, the way to get shapely legs is through this kind of training. One thing you can achieve particularly through glute and quad work is a tight, round bottom, with minimal body fat and no cellulite. As an added benefit, leg training speeds up metabolism, because the glutes and quads make up so much of the body's muscle mass.

At home:

Larry lunges:

Here is a great overall leg exercise, with primary focus in the rear end and the back of the legs. If all you did for you lower body was lunges, then you'd develop great legs. You can do these lunges with dumbbells in your hand, with a barbell on your shoulders, or with no weight at all.

1. Stand with your feet shoulder-width apart and imagine you are on railroad tracks.

2. Step forward on one foot, as if you're taking one giant step forward in the old Simon Says game. When you take the step, your foot should move straight ahead, as if you're walking on a railroad track. Keep your back straight at all times. Do not lean forward.

3. As you step forward, bend your back leg, but never let your knee touch the ground. Then step back and alternate legs.

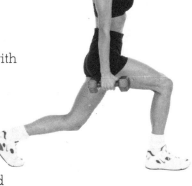

Tips:

- Beginners, do this exercise with no weight.

- If you want to put more emphasis on the muscles in your rear end, when stepping back, lift the toes of your front foot upward and push back on your heel.

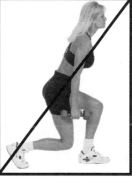

- Keep your legs far enough apart (twelve inches is great). Make sure your back leg goes down far enough when you step forward.

- *Caution:* If you have knee problems, you might want to skip this exercise.

Front Squats:

This is a different kind of squat from what you've seen, because you are going to be putting the bar at the top of your chest, not on your shoulders behind your head. In this exercise, you will be working your thigh muscles and rear end.

1. Hold the bar as if you are going to do an overhead press. (The reason you do this in front is to keep your back straight. it insures proper form and prevents injury.)

2. Stand with your feet shoulder-width apart. (For those of you who are beginners and don't have good flexibility, prop your heels up on a two-by-four.)

3. Then simply pretend you're sitting down. Never let your butt go lower than your knees.

4. When your thighs are parallel to the ground, lift back up—but don't lock the knees at the top of the movement. Keep them slightly bent. And keep your feet flat on the floor at all times.

Tips:

■ When learning this movement, don't use much weight. In fact, you don't even need to use a bar.

■ If your knees bend toward each other and touch during this exercise, you're using too much weight. You will do more reps than usual of this exercise, because you don't need much weight.

- Always keep your hands close to the center of the bar, with your elbows high, and make sure the bar is firmly in place at the top of your chest.

- Avoid using so much weight that your thighs go beyond a parallel position.

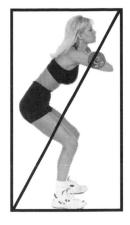

Leg extensions

This exercise, for the front part of the thigh, is a big-time leg shaper, and you can do it without using heavy weight. Just focus on controlling the movement precisely. If you use too much weight, you'll start swinging the weight and lose control.

1. Sit in the leg-extension machine and put your feet behind the pad. Adjust the seat so the pad will hit you right above the foot at the bottom of the ankle.

2. Push up with your legs, flexing your thighs until your legs are nearly straight.

3. Don't come all the way back, because it will put too much stress on the knees. Remember: Safety first.

Tip:

- Keep your back straight against the back pad at all times. Avoid undue pressure and strain on the knees, and keep your legs from going too far back.

Hack squats

For your rear end, and the front and back of your upper legs.

1. Position your back firmly against the pad with your feet about shoulder width apart.

2. Squat down to the point where your butt is parallel to the plat-form.

3. Pushing off your heels while tensing your thigh muscles, lift back up without locking your knees.

Tip:

■ This is not an exercise to do if you have bad knees. The higher you put your heels on the pad, the less strain the exercise puts on your knees.

Leg press

This is another all-over leg exercise. The 45-degree-angle leg press can work the thighs and hips in a way you would not believe.

1. Seated in the angled chair, put your feet on the platform. (The higher your heels are on the platform, the harder you'll work the glute.) Always keep your heels higher than your knees, so as not to put too much strain on the knees.

2. Push up on the platform, and never, never lock your legs.

3. Release the weight and allow it to settle three-quarters of the way back.

Tips:

■ The minute your butt starts to rise up off the seat, you're using too much weight, which puts too much stress on the lower back.

■ Avoid positioning your knees higher than your feet. Avoid allowing the knees to touch; keep the stress on the quads and glutes.

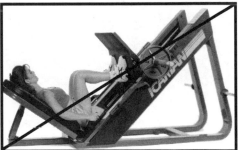

SMALLER MUSCLE GROUPS

■ The smaller muscle groups automatically get worked as you train the larger muscles, and because there's not as much muscle there, you don't have to train them as hard. Of course, I see guys all the time doing a lot of biceps exercises. What they don't know is that they are harming the muscle more than helping it.

For each smaller muscle, I'm only giving you three exercises—one that anyone can perform, followed by one gym exercise, and one advanced exercise. If you're a beginner, you only need to do one of the three.

Triceps

■ The triceps, the muscles along the back of your upper arm, make up two-thirds of that muscle mass, so when you think of developing great arms, you have to concentrate as much on your triceps as you do on your biceps. When fully developed, the triceps make the upper arm look complete. To avoid the old flabby arm syndrome, it makes great sense to keep the triceps as toned and defined as possible. You'll never again be ashamed to wear a sleeveless shirt!

Bench dips

1. With your back
    to the bench,
    put both palms
    on it, keeping
    them close to your body. Extend your
    legs forward until your back is just an inch or
    two from the bench.

2. With your legs slightly bent, lower your butt
    toward the ground.

3. Keeping your back straight the whole time,
    push yourself back to the starting position,
    fully straightening your arms.

Tips :

- As you get stronger,
  you can perform this
  movement with your
  feet up raised on an adjacent bench or chair.

- Don't let your body get
  too far away from the
  bench, and don't do
  this exercise if you
  have bad shoulders.

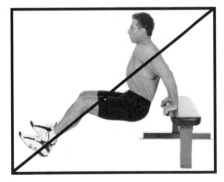

Kickbacks

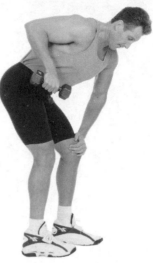

1. With a dumbbell in your hand, bend over so that your torso is parallel to the ground.

2. Raise your elbow so that your triceps are also parallel to the ground.

3. Push the dumbbell backward until your arm is fully extended, flexing your triceps at the top of the movement. Then slowly bring the dumbbell back to where it almost touches the front of your shoulders.

Tip:

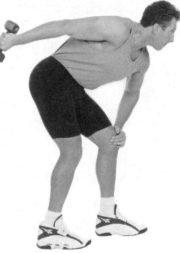

 Watch yourself in a mirror during this exercise to check for form. Try to keep your elbow from swinging.

Push-downs

Another exercise working the entire tricep muscle, push-downs are generally performed on a cable machine with a V-shaped or a straight bar.

1. Standing upright, with your back straight and knees slightly bent, lean a little forward from the waist toward the bar.

2. Push downward, keeping your forearms parallel with one another, and get as full an extension as possible, just short of locking your arms.

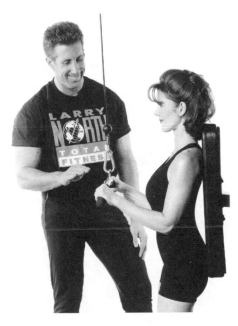 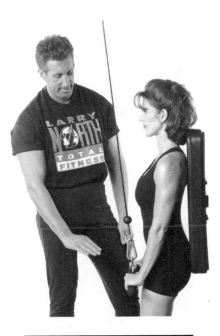

Tip:

- Always keep your elbows pointed out, in front of your body, instead of behind you or to your sides. The right positioning will isolate the tricep muscles.

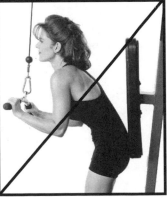

Close-grip bench press

Another complete triceps exercise, this is like the flat-bench chest press, except that you use more weight and keep your hands closer together, just six to eight inches apart. If you're female, start with fifteen pounds; male, forty-five to fifty pounds.

1. Line up the bar at the bottom of the chest, then push straight up, keeping the bar over your chest at all times.

2. Bring the bar to the middle or the lower—not the upper—part of the chest.

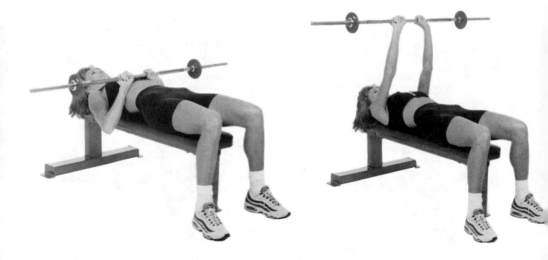

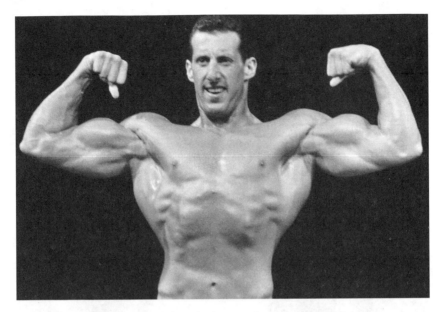

Me, back when I thought I wanted to be a bodybuilder.

Biceps

Biceps, of course, are the arm muscles opposite the triceps that bulge in Charles Atlas ads. But they've come a long way, baby. I think it's great, for instance, that nicely shaped biceps have become so important and sexy for a woman. Again, however, the most common mistake people make in developing biceps is overdoing it. Doing too many sets or using too much weight may bring results, but not without muscle strain and possible loss.

The straight-bar curl

The all-time favorite weight exercise for your biceps. If you're female, start with fifteen pounds, male with thirty to forty pounds.

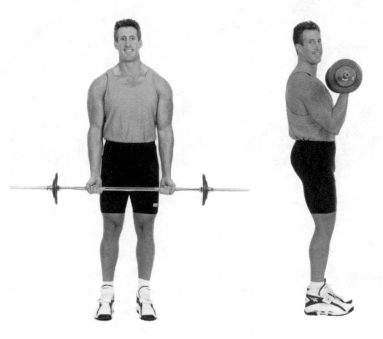

1. Grab the straight bar with your hands closer together than shoulder width.

2. Keeping your arms slightly in front of the body, pull the bar up toward the chin, flex at the top, and then let the bar all the way down to your thighs.

Tips:

■ Your arms must remain parallel with one another, and your elbows should move up only a few inches as you get to the top of the movement.

■ When you start the movement, pretend you're making a muscle, and that will move the bar upward.

■ Keep your back straight, elbows forward, and legs slightly bent. Avoid swinging or jerking the bar up to the chin.

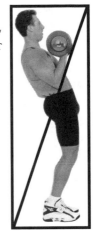

Incline dumbbell curls

1. Sitting on a 45-degree incline bench, put a dumbbell in each hand, and let your arms drop straight down so your hands are directly below your shoulders.

2. With your palms facing away from your body, raise the dumbbells up, making sure to keep your palms up throughout the entire movement (this will isolate the biceps). You don't need to use heavy weights here.

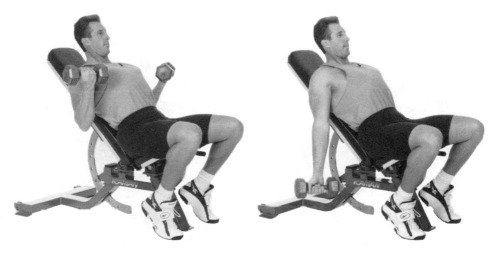

Tip:

■ Keep your elbows in, and make sure your pinkies are higher than your thumbs when you reach the top of the movement.

Forearms

Few people consider working their forearms. But displayed by a short-sleeved shirt, a tight, shapely forearm can be another part of a beautiful, well-toned body. Good forearms are also necessary for numerous daily life functions, from opening jars of food to carrying briefcases and kids. A good forearm is what helps give you a firm, confident handshake. There are two simple exercises to improve your forearms. Again, don't overdo.

At home

Reverse curls

1. Keeping your arms slightly bent in front of your body, pull the bar toward your chin with the palms over the bar.

2. Slowly release the weight and feel the muscle being exercised.

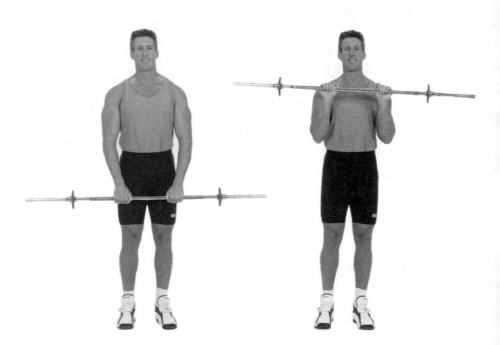

- Your arms must remain parallel, but it's okay if your elbows come forward slightly.

- Lean a little forward, making sure you bring the weight down slowly. Don't let your elbows flap out to the side.

At the gym:

Wrist curls

1. Sit at the end of a bench with dumbbells or a barbell. Lean forward so your forearms are lying on the bench and your wrists hanging over it.

2. Slowly bring the weight all the way down to your finger tips.

3. Roll your fingers around the bar until your wrists curl forward.

Tip:

- Make sure to go down as far as you can, but keep your elbows on the bench at all times.

Hams

■ The hamstring muscles, located directly below the buttocks on the back of the leg, are one of the keys to developing an attractively rounded rear end. When worked properly, your hams look like long muscles on a beautiful racehorse. Regardless of how developed the rest of your lower body is, without adequately toned hamstrings, the lower body doesn't look polished.

At home:

Straight-leg deadlifts

Because there are so few exercises for the hams, I'm only sharing an advanced exercise with you. Be careful. If you do this exercise correctly, you'll develop your hams very quickly. If you do it wrong, you can hurt your lower back. (Remember, if you feel lower back strain at any time, you're doing this movement wrong.)

1. Start by dropping a bar (or even a broomstick), directly in front of you by your thighs, with your hands shoulder-width apart.

2. Bending at the waist, lower the bar to five inches below the knees (less if you can't reach that far). Feel the stretch in your hamstrings.

3. Slowly straighten back up to your starting position.

Tips:

■ As you lower the bar, push your buttocks out in the opposite direction. Despite its name, this movement is not meant to be performed with your legs straight. Do not lock out your knees.

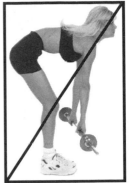

- Keep your shoulders, back, and chest extended the entire time. Don't let your shoulders come forward as you bend forward.

- Avoid a rounded back and locked-out legs, and don't let the bar fall too far below your knees.

At the gym:

Lying down leg curls

1. Lie flat on the leg curl bench and adjust the foot pad so it hits two inches above your heel. Relax the foot at all times.

2. Lift up the pad, making sure you keep lifting until it hits your hamstrings.

3. Release slowly three-quarters of the way.

Tips:

- Keep your toes pointed toward the ceiling.

- Don't use too much weight, or your hips will rotate in the air. Also be careful to limit your range of motion to your legs, because you don't want to cause stress to your lower back.

Hyperextensions

If you are considerably overweight, don't even think about this very advanced movement, for it will hurt the lower back.

1. Lie down on the hyperextension apparatus, with your hands crossed in front of your chest and the back of your feet pushed against the pad.

2. Relax, drop forward, and concentrate on stretching the hamstrings. Don't go all the way down.

3. Lift back up, bringing your shoulders up only so they are parallel to the ground.

Tip:

▪ If you lift up too high, you'll put undue stress on the spine. For this reason, you should perform this movement twice as slowly as you do other movements. And if you have back problems, forget this one.

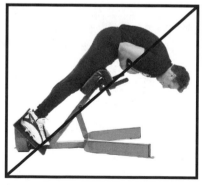

Calves

Your calves are comprised of a stubborn muscle group that doesn't respond to training as rapidly as other body parts, so they tend to get neglected. But think about how important they are. Any time you wear shorts or a dress, you reveal them. A person with developed, nicely toned calves is considered to have good legs, no matter how the rest of the legs look.

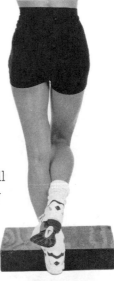

At home:

Single-leg calf raises

1. Standing either on a chair or a low step or flat on the floor—and gripping either a wall or a chair back for balance— wrap one leg gently around the other at the heel.

2. Putting the weight of your body on the ball of the foot that's on the floor, lift your heel as high as you can, like a ballerina.

3. Slowly drop back down, but don't allow your other heel to touch the floor. Repeat, then switch legs.

Tip:

- Perform this exercise slowly, concentrating on a full range of motion.

Standing calf raises

1. Put your feet on the base of the platform of a calf raise machine, dropping your heels off the edge. Separate your feet about four to six inches, toes pointed just slightly inward.

2. Lift your heels as high as you can, then relax as you drop down. At the bottom of the movement, let your heels relax and stretch—and repeat.

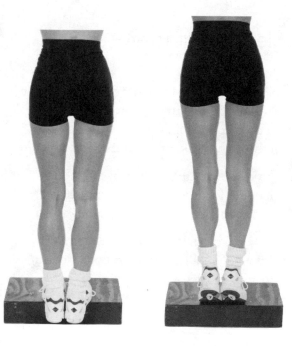

Seated calf raises

1. Using a seated calf machine, perform this exercise the same way you do the standing calf raise, only while sitting down. Standing calf raises work the pretty, upper part of the calf, while the seated calf raise works the area of the calf below.

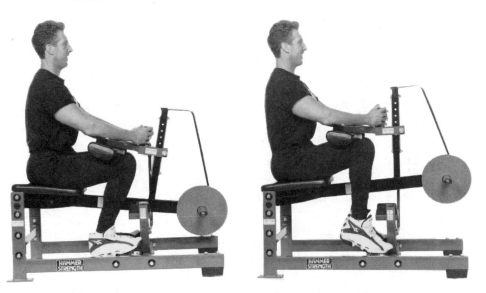

Tips:

-   Concentrate on proper posture and foot position. Avoid performing this exercise too rapidly.

-   Keep your back straight at all times, and avoid using too much weight.

-   Do not continue if your calves cramp.

Abs

If you have a big belly and you think a lot of abdominal exercises will reduce your waistline, forget it. There is no such thing as spot reducing. Sit-ups do not burn the fat around your waist. In fact, there was a study done in which a group of people did 5,000 sit-ups over a period of twenty-seven days. The study found that there was no difference between the amount of fat the individuals lost in the stomach area versus any other part of the body.

Which is not to say you shouldn't tighten the muscles that line your stomach area. After years of training people, I have found out that if you tone and tighten the muscle underneath the fat, you do get an improved appearance. Although you don't lose the fat, you get better definition, because untrained muscle often looks and feels like flab. As you start to develop your body, your abs will become like the focal point of a beautiful picture. Good abs will help you complete the picture of a toned and beautiful body.

For best results, you need to work your abs only two to three times a week. Make sure you work them as you do your other muscle groups, performing the exercises slowly and concentrating so hard that you can only do twenty reps of each ab exercise.

If you can do more than twenty reps, you're not concentrating hard enough. The goal is to develop a rhythm that allows very little rest between sets and exercises. You should only be taking a break of ten to fifteen seconds per set. Why? Since you're not using any weight, you should be able to recover more quickly and move on to the next set.

At home:

Crunches

This is the number-one exercise for working the abs. Note, however, that these are not traditional sit-ups, which can hurt your back.

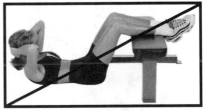

1. Lie flat on your back with your legs propped on a bench or chair. Cross your hands over your chest. (Putting your hands behind your head tends to put too much strain on the neck.)

2. Keep your chin tucked into your chest. Lift your torso at the waist just enough to contract the chest. Keeping your stomach muscles tensed, drop back down to your starting position, but don't touch your back to the ground until you've finished a set of twenty to twenty-five reps.

Tips:

- Instead of keeping your upper back straight, curve and roll into the movement, as if you're rolling a piece of paper into a tube. Keep the shoulders round. Always keeps your tailbone and lower back on the floor, even when you lift up, and do not try to sit all the way up.

- Let the air out of your diaphragm and tighten your stomach muscles at the very beginning of the movement.

- As you become more advanced, you can gradually lift your feet off the bench, holding them a few inches in the air.

Hanging leg raises

These can be performed on a hanging leg apparatus or from a chin-up bar, either by holding the bar or using arm-support straps.

1. Raise your knees upward toward your chest, then slowly drop them back down. Don't swing your legs.

2. Repeat the movement.

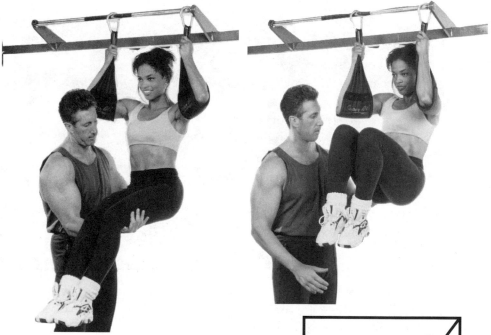

Tip:

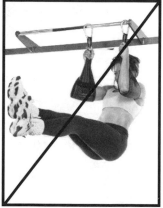

■ Try not to let your heels swing behind your body. If you're a beginner, you might want to do one leg at a time.

Jackknife sit-ups

1. Sit at the end of a flat bench. Put your hands behind you on the bench, close to your buttocks, for balance.

2. Bend your knees to meet the chest, and at the same time bring the chest to meet the knees. The two should meet in the middle of the movement.

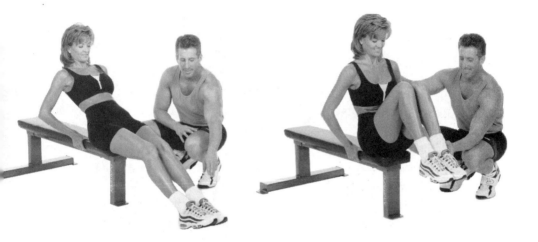

Tips:

- If you're a beginner, keep your legs closer to the floor. As you develop more strength in the midsection, keep raising the angle of your legs.

- Keep your legs together at all times, and avoid leaning too far back. Always perform these reps slowly.

ORDER OF MUSCLE GROUPS

The final thing to think about as you begin your weight training is the order of your routine. You want to train your largest muscle groups first, then proceed to the smaller muscles, because the small body parts are weak links to larger muscle groups. For example, if you work your shoulders before you work your chest and back, you will be so fatigued in your shoulders that you won't be able to get the most out of the chest and back exercises.

For your upper body, start off with your chest, then move on to your back, shoulders, triceps, and then biceps. There is one exception to this general rule. Much later, as you become more advanced, if you encounter a poorly developed body part or one that doesn't respond well to training, work that one first. Why? Because you expend the most energy at the beginning of your workout, and you want to focus greatest intensity on the areas of your body that are most important to you.

If you're male, I recommend you begin your workouts on your upper body parts, then move on to your lower body, because the lower body requires so much energy that you may be too tired to complete your upper body workout. If you're female, I recommend you begin with the lower body, because it's probably a higher priority muscle area for you and you want to use your best energy to develop it.

A Word of Caution

As you begin your training, you may feel in the first two or three weeks that all upper-body exercises are affecting only your arms. In other words, you may not feel that your chest and back are deriving any benefit from your efforts. The reason for this is that your arms are volunteering to do the work, and you're not used to working your chest and back. Don't worry about it. In time, and as you learn what it feels like to focus on these areas, the muscles you're working will show results, too.

A FINAL WORD OF ENCOURAGEMENT

Don't forget the major fact I shared with you at the beginning of this book. The more lean muscle you have, the more active your metabolism will be. And with a higher metabolism, you will burn more fat while at rest.

Conclusion? A weight training program is the main weapon you need to blast away your body fat.

C h a p t e r   N i n e

■ THE ULTIMATE BODY: THE NEXT LEVEL OF YOUR WEIGHT TRAINING PROGRAM

■ Once you get into the program, you'll realize how quickly the body adapts to weight training. Even those of you who do only a few routines will no doubt see some significant changes in your body. But after your first eight weeks, your body might begin to hit a plateau, when you don't feel you're making further progress. Your muscles don't respond, you're fighting boredom, and you

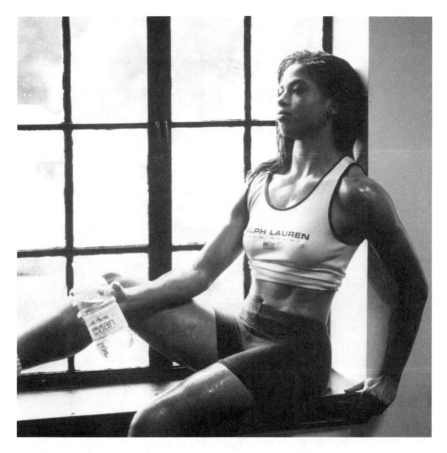

only seem to be going through the motions. That's the ideal time to make subtle changes in parts of your routine.

I'm not talking about anything confusing. Just do what you've always done, only this time also do one or more of the following:

1. Increase the number of reps in each set. Often, that's all it takes to get results again.

2. Change the order of your exercises. For instance, do your incline presses after you do your flat bench flies. If you're a man, do lower-body exercises before the upper-body ones; vice versa if you're a woman.

3. Switch to another exercise for that body part.

4. Decrease the amount of time you rest between each set (but never to less than twenty seconds).

5. Only after you've tried everything else should you try to move on to heavier weights for each exercise. No matter the weight, make sure your technique remains your number-one priority.

Other Plateau Changes

Sometimes, it may not be the weights you need to worry about when you reach your plateau. If you are, for example, losing inches but also strength, you're probably not eating enough. Remember, if you aren't putting the right number of calories into your system, your body will start getting its nutrients from your muscle. Eating too little and exercising too much results in a loss of lean body mass.

However, if you are getting stronger but also expanding around the waist and hips, then you probably need to shave some food off each meal and increase your aerobic activity. Remember, your goal is always to lose inches while increasing strength and energy.

THE FULL-BODY ROUTINE

Want to go for a big workout? Once you're accustomed to all the equipment and you've got your form down, then try this full-body routine. At home or at a gym, you can follow this routine forever and continue to get results. For each exercise listed, complete three sets of ten reps each.

1. Incline barbell press (for your chest)

2. Flat bench flies (chest)

3. One-arm dumbbell row (back)

4. Bent-over row (back)

5. Upright row (shoulders)

6. Side lateral raises (shoulders)

7. Bench dips (triceps)

8. Straight bar curls (biceps)

9. Lunges (quads and glutes)

10. Front squats (quads and glutes)

11. Straight-leg deadlifts (hams)

12. Single-leg calf raises (calves)

13. Crunches (abs)

A Split Routine

I also want to introduce you to a routine that I've taught a lot of people, with wonderful results. It's a three-day-a-week routine that many people follow once they move into the intermediate stages of their training

On day one, train only your upper body. The very next day, train only your lower body. Then—you earned it!—take two complete days of rest. On day five, do a full-body workout. Take days six and seven off. Then start all over again.

With this split routine, you end up doing an increased amount of work, because you exercise fewer body parts at a higher intensity in each workout. In the end, you do three exercises (instead of the usual two) for each major muscle group. (You'll still complete two to three sets.) For the smaller muscle groups, do two exercises instead of the usual one.

A note to those of you working out at home: If you don't have the machines or the additional equipment needed for the split routine, simply add sets for both your larger and smaller muscle groups. Here's the program:

Day One—Upper Body

Do two to three sets, ten reps each.

1. Incline barbell presses (chest)

2. Flat bench flies (chest)

3. Pec deck (chest)

4. One-arm dumbbell rows (back)

5. Bend-over rows (back)

6. Lat pull-downs (back)

7. Upright rows (shoulders)

8. Side lateral raises (shoulders)

9. Overhead presses (shoulders)

10. Bench dips (triceps)

11. Push-downs (triceps)

12. Straight bar curl (biceps)

13. Incline dumbbell curls (biceps)

Day Two—Lower Body

You'll do the same two to three sets per exercise, but increase the reps from ten to twelve or fifteen. You need to increase the number of reps because of the reduction in exercises and because the lower body tends to require more reps to get desired results.

1. Larry lunges (quads and glutes)

2. Front squats (quads and glutes)

3. Leg presses (quads and glutes)

4. Straight-leg deadlifts (hams)

5. Leg curls (ham)

6. Single-leg calf raises (calves)

7. Seated calf raises (calves)

8. Crunches (abs)

9. Jackknife sit-ups (abs)

Days Three and Four—Rest

Day Five — Full Body

On this day, do your traditional full-body routine, but increase your repetitions from ten to twelve.

1. Incline barbell presses (chest)
2. Flat bench flies (chest)
3. One-arm dumbbell rows (back)
4. Bent-over rows (back)
5. Upright rows (shoulders)
6. Side lateral raises (shoulders)
7. Bench dips (triceps)
8. Straight bar curls (biceps)
9. Lunges (quads and glutes)
10. Straight-leg deadlifts (hams)
11. Single-leg calf raises (calves)
12. Crunches (abs)

Days Six and Seven — Rest

The Four-Day Split

If you've really gotten into the program and enjoy being in the gym more than three times a week, try the four-day split.

Again, heed this warning: a four-day routine is the most work you should ever do. Unless you're a competitive athlete or bodybuilder, never work more than four days a week. Here's the traditional four-day split:

Day One — Upper Body

Day Two — Lower Body

Day Three — Rest

Day Four—Upper Body

Day Five—Lower Body

Day Six and Day Seven—Rest

The Four-Day Split Routine, Part 2

Sometimes during a four-day routine, you work parts of your lower and upper body on the same day. Such a routine constantly challenges your body by expecting something new from it. Day one and day three, you'll work your chest, shoulders, triceps, hams, and back. On day two and day four, you'll work your back, biceps, quads, and calves. In this routine, we will occasionally increase the number of sets and reps:

Day One

Chest:
1. Incline presses—three sets, ten to twelve reps

2. Dips—three sets, ten reps

3. Flat bench flies—three sets, twelve reps

4. Pec deck—two sets, fifteen reps

Shoulders:
1. Overhead presses—two to three sets, twelve reps

2. Side lateral raises—three sets, ten to twelve reps

3. Upright rows—two to three sets, eight to ten reps

4. Bent-over lateral raises—two sets, twelve reps

Triceps:
1. Push-downs—three sets, twelve to fifteen reps

2. Bench dips—four sets, eight to twelve reps

Hams:
1. Lying-down leg curls—four sets, twelve reps

2. Straight-leg deadlifts—two to three sets, ten to twelve reps

Day Two

Back:
1. Lat pull-downs (using a wide grip)—three sets, eight to ten reps

2. Bent-over rows—three sets, eight to ten reps

3. Lat pull-downs (closed grip)—two to three sets, eight to twelve reps

4. Pull-ups—two to three sets, six to ten reps

Biceps:
1. Straight bar curls—three sets, ten to twelve reps

2. Incline dumbbell curls—three sets, ten to twelve reps

Quads:
1. Leg extensions—three to four sets, twelve to fifteen reps

2. Leg presses—three to four sets, twelve to twenty reps

3. Front squats—three sets, twelve reps

Calves:
1. Seated calf raises—two to three sets, fifteen to twenty reps

2. Standing calf raises—two to three sets, twelve to fifteen reps

Day Three—Rest

Day Four—Repeat Day One

Day Five—Repeat Day Two

Day Six and Seven—Rest

For Women Only

I know some of you are finding these advanced routines a bit intimidating. Just for you, I've devised a great three-day-a-week advanced routine that hits every body part and allows you to develop your muscles without making them big.

Day One

Chest:
1. Incline dumbbell presses—two to three sets, ten reps

2. Pec deck—two to three sets, ten reps

Shoulders:
1. Overhead presses

2. Side lateral raises—two sets, ten reps

3. Bent-over lateral raises—two sets, ten reps

Triceps:
Push-downs—three sets, ten to twelve reps

Legs:
1. Leg presses—three sets, twelve to fifteen reps

2. Hyperextensions—three sets, twelve to fifteen reps

3. Leg curls—three sets, twelve to fifteen reps

Day Two

Back:
1. Lat pull-downs (using wide grip)—three sets, ten to twelve reps

2. Lat pull-downs (using close grip)—three sets, ten to twelve reps

Biceps:
Curls (using dumbbells or barbell)—three sets, ten to twelve reps

Legs:
1. Leg extensions—three to four sets, ten to twelve reps

2. Front squats—three sets, ten to twelve reps

3. Larry lunges—three to four sets, ten to twelve each leg

4. Standing calf raises—four to five sets, fifteen to twenty reps

Days Three and Four—Rest

Day Five

Legs only:
1. Leg extensions—three sets, ten to twenty reps

2. Leg presses—three sets, ten to twenty reps

3. Larry lunges—three sets, ten to twenty reps

4. Lying leg curls—three sets, ten to twenty reps

5. Hyperextensions—three sets, ten to twenty reps

6. Seated calf raises—three sets, ten to twenty reps

7. Standing calf raises—three sets, ten to twenty reps

Days Six and Seven—Rest

Weak Areas

As you progress, you're likely to feel that one body part might not be in shape compared to the rest of your body. If this happens, you may want to go into the gym and work that body part alone. By now, you're knowledgeable enough to select any number of exercises to refine your problem area. Here are a few examples of problem area routines:

Better butt routine:
1. Lying down leg curls—three sets, twelve reps

2. Leg presses—three sets, fifteen to twenty reps

3. Straight-leg dead lifts—two to three sets, ten to twelve reps

4. Hyperextensions—two to three sets, ten to fifteen reps

5. Larry lunges—two to three sets, ten reps (for each leg)

Biceps blast:
1. Straight bar curls—three sets, ten reps

2. Incline dumbbell curls—three sets, twelve to fifteen reps

Head-turner legs:
1. Leg extensions—three to five sets, twelve to fifteen reps

2. Front squats—four sets, twenty reps

3. Leg curls—three sets, fifteen reps

4. Straight-leg deadlifts—three sets, twelve reps

5. Larry lunges—five sets, ten reps

6. Standing calf raises—five sets, twelve to twenty reps

The "I've got to get big" routine:
Skip this section unless you're really advanced and want big muscles. This routine is for those advanced weight trainers who are dead set on gaining size. Over five days of training, you'll focus on particular body parts, and you'll do lots of sets. On the last training day of the week, you'll do a light upper-body pump, in which you'll reduce the weight you're lifting and work on the weaker upper-body muscles. This is my favorite routine to increase strength and build muscles. You'll see a few new exercises added to the routine on some days.

Day One—
Chest and Front Delts

1. Bench press—three to four sets, eight to twelve reps

2. Incline dumbbell press—three to four sets, eight to twelve reps

3. Dips—three to four sets, eight to twelve reps

4. Flat bench flies—three to four sets, eight to twelve reps

5. Pec deck—two to three sets, twelve to fifteen reps

6. Front lateral raises (like side lateral raises, except you raise your dumbbells one at a time in front of you to shoulder height)

Day Two—Back

1. Pull-ups—three to four sets, eight to ten reps

2. Bent-over rows—three to four sets, eight to ten reps

3. Lat pull-downs (wide grip)—three sets, eight to ten reps

4. One-arm dumbbell rows—two sets, eight to ten reps

5. Machine rows—three to four sets, eight to ten reps

6. Shrugs (holding a barbell, with your arm straight down at your side, move only your shoulders straight up toward your ears, then release slowly)

Day Three— Bi's, Tri's and Side Delts

1. Pick any three biceps exercises—three sets, ten to twelve reps

2. Pick any three triceps exercises—three sets, eight to twelve reps

3. Side lateral raises—five sets, ten to twelve reps

Day Four—Legs

1. Leg extensions—three to four sets, ten to twenty reps

2. Leg presses—three sets, ten to twenty reps

3. Front squats—three to four sets, ten to twenty reps

4. Larry lunges—three sets, ten to twenty reps

5. Leg curls—three sets, ten to twenty reps

6. Straight-leg deadlifts—three sets, ten to twenty reps

7. Standing calf raises—four sets, ten to twenty reps

8. Seated calf raises—four sets, ten to twenty reps

Day Five—Rest

Day Six—
Light Upper Body Pump

1. Flat bench flies—three sets, twelve reps

2. Incline dumbbell presses—three sets, twelve reps

3. Pec deck—two sets, twelve reps

4. Pull-ups—two to three sets, ten reps

5. Upright rows—two to three sets, ten reps

6. Straight bar curls—two to four sets, eight to twelve reps

7. Incline dumbbell curls—two to three sets, twelve reps

8. Triceps push-downs—three to five sets, twelve to fifteen reps

Day Seven—Rest

One-Body-Part-Per-Day Routine

No matter what I say, there's going to be the die-hard weightlifter who decides to go to the gym every day. All right, if you insist, then try a program in which you work only one body part per day. Do many exercises for that one body part, then leave it alone for a week. For each large muscle, do four to five exercises, as many as three sets per exercise. For a smaller muscle, do three to four exercises, two to three sets per exercise. Here's an example:

Day one: chest—five exercises, three sets each, eight to fifteen reps per set

Day two: back—four to five exercises, three sets, eight to twelve reps

Day three: shoulders—four exercises, three sets, eight to ten reps

Day four: biceps—four exercises, two to three sets, eight to ten reps

Day five: triceps—four exercises, two to three sets, eight to fifteen reps

Day six: quads—five exercises, three sets, eight to twenty reps

Day seven: hams—four exercises, two to three sets, twelve to twenty reps

Day eight: calves—four exercises, two to three sets, twelve to twenty reps

I don't recommend one body part per day as a regular routine, but if you feel you've reached a difficult plateau and need a change for a week or so, give it a try.

Most Advanced

Once you are fully into the program, far past the beginner's phase, you'll want to try more techniques. The following are ideas for varying your routines, but they should only be incorporated once every four to five workouts.

1. *Forced reps.* When your muscles wear down during an exercise and you can no longer perform a rep on your own, have someone assist you lifting the weight for one or two additional reps. More than two is a waste of time and can cause injury.

2. *Super sets.* Super setting means doing more than one exercise without any rest in between. After a few straight exercises, then you rest. You can super set the same body part—such as combining flat bench flies with incline presses. Or you can super set unrelated body parts—such as incline presses with lat pull-downs. You shouldn't try super sets for the first three months of your workouts,

but later, if you want to increase the intense focus on certain muscles, this is one way to do it.

3. *Training until positive failure.* With this technique, you start a set and keep going until you can no longer move the weight. Clearly, this is an intense training technique, one that shouldn't be used routinely. Weight training should be fun—not draining, painful, or downright dangerous.

4. *Slow motion training.* Using this technique, you take two seconds to pull the weight down and four seconds to release it back to the starting position. This is a good way to teach you to focus on the muscle group you're training. But beware of performing every set in slo-mo, because it will put too much stress on your joints.

5. *Iso-tension training.* Squeeze and hold the weight at the top of the movement for a period of time, then slowly release. With leg extensions, for example, hold the weight at the top of the movement until you feel a burn, then let it back down.

Final Suggestions

It doesn't hurt, as you become more advanced, to overhaul your routine every six to twelve weeks, sometimes even going back to a beginner routine for a while. I'd even suggest taking a week off every three months, because you never want to push your body to the point where it simply burns out and becomes vulnerable to injury.

As much as I've made fun of the musclehead mentality of weight rooms, you can actually learn a lot by leafing through muscle and bodybuilding magazines. You'll find a useful variety of other routines and other movements. But remember, these are routines done by champion bodybuilders who practically live in the weight room and eat up to 6,000 calories per day. If you try to follow all their routines, you'll overtrain and burn yourself out. Never make your routine feel like work. If it's not enjoyable, then you need to lighten up.

One way to stay motivated and enjoy yourself is to train with a workout partner. A partner can pay close attention to your routines, correct your form, and inspire you when you feel like leaving the gym. Ultimately, of course, the will to continue must come from within. I know you have that will. Now that you have the right tools for life, there's only one thing left to do—stick with the program!

ELONGATING THE MUSCLE: STRETCHING EXERCISES FOR A LEAN BODY

Sure, I used to hate to stretch. I always wondered, "Is this really helping my body?"

What I have since discovered is that for those doing this program, especially those starting out, stretching can be as important as lifting weights. You have to stretch to avoid the contracted, muscle-bound look. You want to elongate your muscle, and that's only going to happen if you stretch.

One of the best ways to avoid soreness or injury is to do some basic stretching exercises at the end of a workout, when your muscles are warm. (You can even do some of these stretches while you're resting between weight training exercises.)

Using the right stretching exercises, you're giving your muscles a chance to relax and releasing body tension. Moreover, stretching will help shape your body. Your posture will improve, and you will gain greater mobility and flexibility. Instead of being the kind of weightlifter who cannot bend over and touch your toes, you will cultivate a beautifully lean, limber appearance.

In this chapter, I'll share with you a variety of stretches from which to choose. You don't have to do them all each day. Do a couple of upper body stretches one day and a few lower body the next. The good news is that you don't have to stretch for very long—no more than ten to twenty seconds per stretch. It's a myth that you need to stay in a painful stretching position for minutes at a time to gain benefit.

But always remember to stretch smoothly. Never bounce or make any movement that hurts. If you cannot touch your toes in a stretch, that's fine. Stretch as far as you can, and eventually the muscle fibers will lengthen even more. And, most important: Remember to breathe while you are stretching.

Inhale and exhale deeply as you stretch in each position. Count to three as you inhale and exhale. After getting the hang of the time interval, you will not even have to count. As you inhale, think of relaxing the muscle group, and as you exhale, think of elongating the muscle area. Breathing is very important, because it uses a natural body rhythm to stretch muscles like elastic bands. If you just pull and pull a muscle, it will give only so much. Releasing and relaxing in between will deepen the stretch.

Full Body Stretch

Lie on your back with your feet flat about eighteen inches from your hips. Relax your arms down by your sides. Stay in this position for a few moments, breathing effortlessly. Let your spine be heavy and rest flat on the floor. Stay in this position and let the tension melt out of your back and limbs. Imagine your body expanding beyond its limits.

Next, gently straightening one leg at a time, clasp your hands together over your head and pull your shoulders away from your body like taffy. Breathe in and out naturally. Gently flex your ankles by inching your heels away from and your toes toward your body. Hold for ten to twenty seconds. Repeat.

Full Body Stretch, version 2

Get into the full body stretch position described. Interlock your hands underneath your head. Bring your left leg over the right leg and gently press the right leg to the floor. Hold for ten to twenty seconds. Repeat on the other side. It is imperative that you keep your elbows, head, and shoulders flat on the floor. Exhale as you press your leg to the floor.

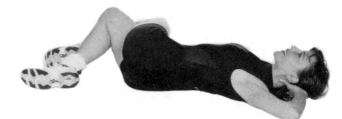

Full Body Stretch, version 3

While standing, put your hands together and bring them straight up above your head. Hold for ten to twenty seconds. Then gently lower your arms. Think of stretching your hands as far away from your feet as possible. Lengthen the spine vertically. Don't stick your chest or buttocks out or lower or raise your chin. Instead, think of your navel as touching your spine. This visualization will help make your abdominals work more effectively.

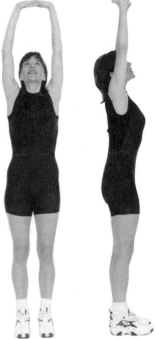

Neck Stretch

Put the palm of your hand on the top of your head and gently bend your head forward. Breathe and hold the stretch for twenty seconds. Return your head to its natural position, then put your right hand on the left side of your head and gently pull your head toward your right shoulder. Your ear should be parallel to your shoulder, but not touching it. Then sense the stretch along the left side of your neck and hold it as you breathe.

Return your head to its natural position and switch hands, then repeat on the opposite side. This is a simple but important releasing stretch, because in weightlifting, you unconsciously build a lot of tension in your neck.

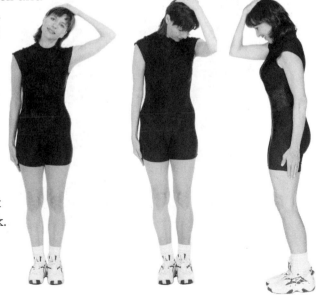

Shoulder Stretch

First, simply inhale and raise your shoulders to your ears—then breathe out and drop your shoulders. Follow up with simple shoulder rolls, circling your shoulders forward and then backward.

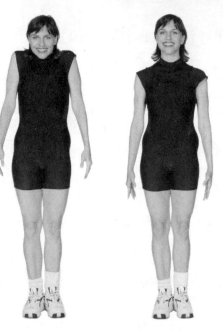

Deltoid Stretch

For a more specific shoulder stretch, reach your left arm across your body below your right shoulder. Use your right hand to grab your left wrist and pull it toward your body. To maximize the stretch, keep your left shoulder still (the tendency is to let your body move right). Next, place your left hand on your right shoul-

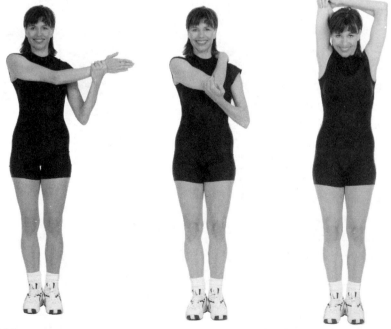

der as if you are patting yourself on your back. Cup your left elbow with your right hand. Pull your elbow back toward your right shoulder.

Finally, point the left elbow toward the ceiling. With your right hand, pull your left elbow toward the center of your back. Repeat on the opposite side. Hold all stretches ten to twenty seconds.

Pectoral Stretch

Stand directly facing the wall, an arm's length away. Put your arm at shoulder level against the wall, press your hand against the wall, and move your body back, shifting your feet in little steps, until you can't go any farther without losing a grip on the wall. Keep your arm extended, but do not lock your elbows, and hold for ten to twenty seconds.

Walk yourself back around to the starting position. Repeat with the other arm. You will feel a great stretch right across the chest, as well as getting a partial deltoid and bicep stretch.

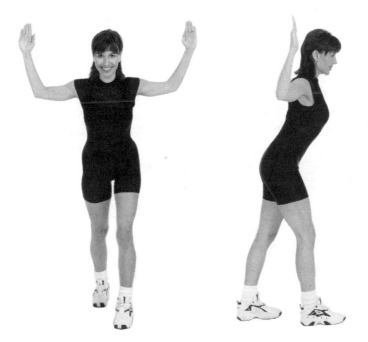

Side Stretch

Standing with your feet at shoulder-width apart, raise your left arm over your head and then bend your body to the right, keeping your shoulders in front of your hips. Think of extending your body out into space. Rather than contracting the right side of your body, think of lengthening both sides as much as you can. Always keep your arm anchored against the side of your head. Breathe and stretch for ten to twenty seconds. Return and reverse to the other side.

Lower Back Stretch

Lie on your back with both feet on the floor, your knees sticking straight up. Bring your right knee up until it's resting on your body. Put your hands below your kneecap, pull, and inhale deeply. As you exhale, gently pull your leg closer to your body. As you inhale, allow your right leg to return to its resting position on your chest. Repeat four times. Think of lengthening your lower back as you deepen the flexion of your right hip socket. Return your right leg to the floor and stretch the opposite side. This stretch is great for anyone with back pain, especially sciatic problems.

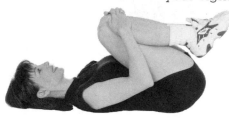

Feet and Lower Leg Stretch

Sit with your legs extended in front of your body. Keep your legs slightly bent, with your knees pointed straight at the ceiling. Gently point your feet away from your body. Then push your heels away from your body while flexing your feet toward your body. Repeat ten times. Now, rotate your feet in a circle ten times in one direction, then reverse direction. While circling, try to spread your toes as far apart as possible, but do not move your kneecaps.

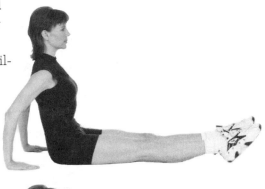

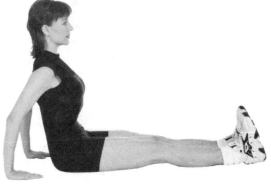

Next, pull your right foot toward your left hip with both hands. Turn the sole of your foot to the ceiling. Hold this position for ten to twenty seconds. Try to pull the tops of your toes into your left shoulder to increase your stretch. Then put your heel on the floor and pull your toes back toward your knee. Hold each position for ten to twenty seconds. Repeat with your left foot.

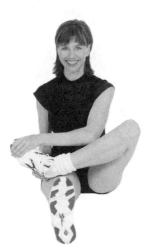

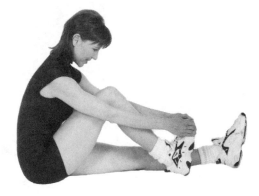

Hamstring Stretch

Lie flat on the floor with one leg against the floor, and point the other leg toward the ceiling, creating an L shape. Your body should be as close to the floor as possible, but it is equally important to keep your hips aligned. Hold this position for twenty seconds. Breath naturally and let the weight of your leg sink into the floor.

Alternative Hamstring Stretch

Kneel on one knee while holding onto a piece of equipment or furniture, or touching the ground. Align your body, making sure your feet are pointed directly ahead. Your knees must be directly in line with your feet, and your hips must be squared. Now straighten both legs. Breathe in and out naturally. Repeat with the other leg.

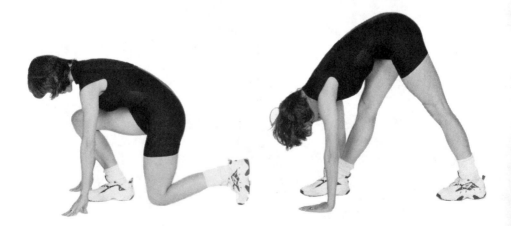

Lower Body Stretch

Sit with your back very straight, knees bent and your feet flat on the floor. Clasp your hands behind your head. Twist your body to the right, and extend your left elbow to the floor while your right elbow points toward the ceiling. Return to your starting position, twist to the other side, and aim your right elbow toward the floor. Repeat three times for each side. Do not let your hips rock from side to side, and keep your hips and feet firmly planted on the floor. Breathe out as you twist. If there is any pain in your lower back, stop and try again later, without as much torque in your twist.

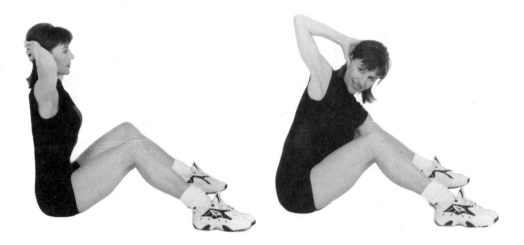

Quadricep Stretch

Stand tall with your feet directly underneath you. Place one leg on a chair behind you. Keep your knee directly underneath your hip; do not let it wander outside the hip. Make sure you're stretching in your hip joint. Then, keeping the exact form, use your hand to pull your heel toward your rear end. Remember to keep your stomach pulled against your spine and your knee in line with your hip. Do not arch your back.

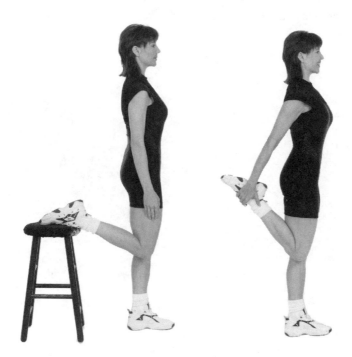

Advanced Quadricep Stretch

Start in a standing position. Bring your right foot back directly behind your hip, and place your right knee on the floor. Place both hands on your left knee. Keep your body straight, your head aligned with your shoulders, and your shoulders aligned with your hips. Pull your stomach in toward your backbone. Repeat with your other leg. If you feel any pain in the lower back region, lean forward slightly.

Overall Body Stretch, Focusing on Hip, Waist and Back

While sitting upright on the floor, bring your right leg across your left leg and slide your heel toward your rear end. Reach over your right leg with your left arm, and hug the leg to your body. Bring your elbow in front of your knee to increase the stretch. Hold this position as you push back with your left arm. Look over your right shoulder, (if this is too difficult, hug your knee to your chest and work up to a twisting action.)

Come out of the twist. Let your right knee relax, and round forward with your palms on the floor. Hold ten to twenty seconds.

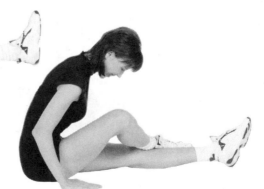

Now, return to an upright sitting position on the floor and push your left hip directly over your right hip, so your body is facing sideways. Place your left foot on the floor by your right knee. (Keep your navel lined up with your spine.) With your ribs in and your body relaxed, hold the stretch for ten to twenty seconds. Switch legs. (To make this more difficult, keep both legs together.)

Roll to your abdomen. Support your body weight on your elbows while you lift your head. Hold this position to stretch the front of your body.

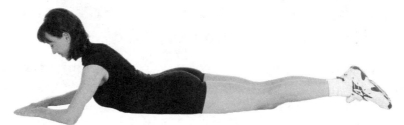

Lie on your back and bend both knees. Bring your right ankle on top of your left knee. Use both hands to support your left thigh as you lift it toward you and hold. Repeat movement on the other side.

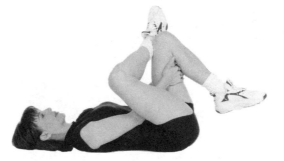

Now lie on your back and bring the soles of your feet together. Spread out your knees and point them toward opposite sides of the room. Hold, and relax.

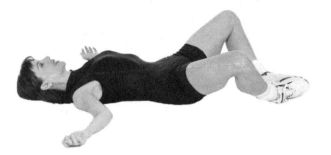

Chapter Eleven

THE NORTH BODY: THE FINAL STEP TO YOUR LEANEST BODY

So here you are, on the last chapter of this book. At this point, one of two things is happening. Either (A) You are totally pumped up, leaping for joy that you've finally learned how to break out of the old diet and fitness patterns, or (B) You still aren't sure you want to embrace a new program.

I know many of you have convinced yourselves that you have legitimate "reasons" you can't get involved in a program such as mine. For years, I've listened to people explain their reasons to me. "I work twelve hours a day." "I have three kids." "I haven't exercised in twenty years." "I need to lose some weight before I work out." "I used to be a good athlete, but now I have bad knees." "I have heart disease." "Everyone in my family is overweight and always has been, so who would I be fooling?"

I don't mean to be rude, but I simply refuse to listen to excuses. "Oh, please, Larry," I remember one client saying to me. "It's easy for you to act righteous. Fitness is what you do for a living. You don't understand what our lives are like."

I'm sorry, but I know far more than many of you what a life of excuses is like. I know firsthand the depression that can set in when you are driven by fear of failure, when you are hesitant to release the ambition inside you. All of us are filled with this wonderful power inside us. The question is, can we find the strength to unleash it?

At the beginning of this book, I wrote about my mother and her lifelong struggle to lose weight. Now I want to tell you about my father and what I learned from him. I have never seen anyone work harder at becoming a failure than my father. He failed in every single thing he did in his life. He failed at school, dropping out in the seventh grade. He could never keep a job. He failed in his marriages. He failed as a father. A compulsive gambler who was constantly losing money, he was arrested dozens of times for everything from bank fraud to mail fraud.

Eventually, he became famous for his failures. In the 1970s, the CBS news program *60 Minutes* did a long story featuring my father as a typical gambling addict. I was just a young, overweight teenager then. In one scene, I was shown with my father at a race track, watching him gamble away the family's entire savings. I often stare at that piece of footage. I am sitting beside him, my face a jumble of emotions. It's clear that I desperately care for him, and at the same time, I am desperately afraid. Here was my father—a funny, charming man, a man with a very high IQ—whose life was spiraling out of control in front of my very eyes. When he'd lost the money at the race track (which he inevitably did), he'd wink at me and say, "Don't worry, I've got a way to get it back." To show his love for me, he'd take me to a fancy restaurant, where he'd order a wildly expensive meal. Then, no matter how much money he had in his pocket, he'd walk out on the check and head off that night to an all-night craps game. If he didn't win there, he'd find a loan shark to lend him $100 so he could start all over the next day.

Of course, my mother had to work nonstop to earn money to pay the rent and feed me and my two brothers. More than once, my father stole money out of her pocketbook. As part of one of his sentencings, he was sent to a gambling center to get better, but once there, he taught five of the people in his therapy group how to swindle banks. During an outpatient day, he took them all to the race track.

My father always thought there was going to be some magical stroke of fate that would change his life—the winning lotto number or a victory at the track. But the more time that passed, the more he lost his way. When *60 Minutes* returned to visit my father in 1986 for a follow-up story, correspondent Harry Reasoner asked him if he had any regrets. My father tearfully broke down and said, "Well, I regret losing my family. I regret being in prison." Then he suddenly smiled and said, "Other than that, I don't have any regrets." When I heard that response, it was as if someone had knocked me over the head with a sledgehammer. Here was his chance to admit his failure and move forward. But anybody watching knew that if he had the chance to live his life again, he would choose to do exactly what he'd done before.

ESCAPING FROM FAILURE

Why am I telling my father's story in a fitness book? It's very simple. The great tragedy of his life was that he never knew how to get himself back on course. As the years passed, it only became easier for him to remain a failure. He worked hard at being a failure—he was at the track or the casinos day and night trying to win money. He never understood that he worked harder at being a failure than most people do at being a success. If he'd only been able to stay focused on success, he would have reached his potential and found happiness that he never thought were possible.

Through my father, I learned how quickly and easily anyone, including myself, could become a failure. But as I watched him fail over and over, I also made a decision—a very simple decision—that I would never do the same thing.

Today I know what it takes to live a life without excuses. When I decided to open my first gym, I had no money. I didn't even have a bank account. But I was not going to take no for an answer. The day I went to the bank to get a loan, the skies opened up and a drenching downpour hit Dallas. I was in an old car with a leaky sunroof that collapsed under the weight of the water. I was soaking wet, wearing the only suit I owned. I looked like an idiot. But I went ahead and walked into that bank and said to the banker, "This dream of mine is going to happen." I never stopped believing I could be successful.

You may think I acted that way because my personality is different from yours. No. I had to learn to believe in myself. And you know what? It's not that hard. I visualized what I wanted to do—seeing truly is believing—and I convinced myself that my goals were going to become a reality. You can do the same thing by setting goals for your body. The minute you visualize the body you want, you're on your way to success. Don't lose that picture of who you want to be.

Let me give you an example of someone who believed in a new image of himself. In Dallas, there's an accountant named Gary Hotchkiss, who owns a successful firm and lectures on financial topics around the country. For two years, he listened to my radio show, taking in all my information on proper nutrition and exercise. Finally, he worked up the courage to make an appointment with me for a consultation.

When I first met him, I couldn't believe what I was seeing. Gary Hotchkiss weighed 445 pounds. He barely fit through my office door. He took a look around at the fit people working out in the gym, and then he sat precariously on a chair.

I listened to him tell me about his past diets. On one diet, he said, he lost fifty pounds in two months—only to gain it all back soon after. Other instructors, he told me, had ordered him not to exercise because they were afraid he'd get hurt or that his heart wouldn't be able to take it. Indeed, when I put him on a treadmill, he couldn't go for five minutes on even the lowest speed. He was so out of breath that he could barely take another step. He couldn't use any of the weight machines in the gym because he couldn't fit into them!

To almost everyone in the gym, Gary's situation seemed hopeless. They thought that maybe the North program could take him down quite a few pounds, but what real difference would it make? Instead of weighing 445 pounds, he'd weigh 345 pounds. Who would notice?

Yet I took a deep breath and said, "Gary, there's a lean man inside waiting to get out." He paused, and he said, "I know there is, Larry." My eyes filled with tears. He had a picture of himself as he wanted to be. Right then, I vowed that I was going to do everything I could to help him get that lean man out.

Of course, I wasn't the key to his success. It was his own desire to change. He wanted to escape from a life of failure. He started eating small, low-fat meals six times a day. He didn't starve himself. He did what it took to make sure he kept the fat out of his diet. He learned to special order in restaurants. He learned to prepare healthy nonfat meals. He began a modest weight training program and was soon carrying a set of dumbbells with him on the road when he traveled on business. Often when he was out of town, he'd look up a gym in the Yellow Pages and go work out there. He also began a simple walking program, because he realized he could walk no matter where he was. Within eight weeks, he was walking 45 minutes a day. Soon after that, he was walking for an hour a day.

Gary Hotchkiss's body changed—permanently. In his first seven months on the program, he lost 190 pounds. Today, five years after starting the program, he has kept thirty-four inches off his waist and has stayed comfortably at 218 pounds.

Now here's the message that should remain emblazoned on your brain. Gary Hotchkiss did nothing more than what is in this book. He did nothing more than what I'm asking you to do. He made some alterations in his eating habits and took an hour a day to get in his workouts—and he demolished his body fat.

Why was he able to do it? Because he believed in a leaner, healthier version of himself!

My father always used to tell me that life at its best was a fierce struggle. He was wrong. Gary Hotchkiss will tell you that life is a beautiful thing, that every single thing about it can be cherished to its fullest. His new body didn't come through a fierce struggle. It was developed with a very simple program, one that gave him the self-esteem and comfort that he'd never before known in his life. He learned that success does not always come from working harder than everyone else. It comes from working smarter. And that, my friends, is the essence of the Larry North Program.

PROGRESS, NOT PERFECTION

I'll be very honest about the North Program. Perfection is an impossibility. Progress is what's important. And I'm talking here about slow, steady progress. I know this sounds sacrilegious compared to the language of every other self-help book that you've read, but if you're looking for immediate perfection, you're going to fail. As I learned from my father's life, there is no such thing as an overnight success. Sudden reversals of fortune are never real.

If you understand this distinction—between the desire for steady progress and the desire for instant perfection—then it's much easier to stay on the program. With the North Program, there is no finish line. The fact is, you can't make permanent changes in your body quickly, and if you just recognize that fact, you'll take a lot of pressure off yourself.

Because I don't focus on perfection as a goal, I have included a modified version of the program and allow "cheat" meals. The problem with demanding perfection is that it's too easy to quit when you don't achieve it. You'll think, "Well, maybe I should try another program." And when you fail at that one, you'll move on to something else.

It's important that you don't view the North Program as an attempt to make you undergo a major life-style change. Most people hate the idea of having to make "life-style" changes. I simply want you to change some habits. The North Program is a system of replacing bad habits with good ones: eating more meals properly, performing less strenuous cardiovascular exercise for longer periods, and training with weights two to three times a week. As I have said before, this isn't a pass-fail program. You can follow 50 percent of this program and still get results.

The Inevitable Setback

Having said all that, I know that even if you jump wholeheartedly on the bandwagon, you're still likely to suffer a setback. You're going to get involved in the North Program, work hard at it, and then—for various reasons—begin to back away. You'll feel as if you've lost your motivation to get lean.

Everyone is going to have setbacks. I know that. I have them, too. But we shouldn't let them upset us or stand in the way of our progress, especially when they're relatively minor. In fact, the key to staying successful is learning how to rebound from our setbacks.

Let's take the example of a woman I know who's really been working out and eating correctly. She's making a lot of progress. Compared to a year ago, her body is so different—shapelier, leaner, more powerful, stunningly attractive. She feels a fresh burst of excitement every day. Her life is turning around. But what happens? She starts sliding away from the program! She slows down. She thinks, "Oh, well, there's no way I can go back to the old body. Look how far I've come."

Humans are a strange bunch. It seems that once we get what we want, we stop wanting it. Moreover, in physical fitness, once we get just close to what we want, somehow we think we're through. I think about how many people I've watched who do what it takes to get in shape. I've seen people who have gone through fantastic weight loss, whose stomachs have gone from pot bellies to nearly flat bellies. But then they stop.

It happens over and over. People get to the crest of the hill, and almost without knowing it, they stop climbing. They think they don't have to watch their food consumption as closely. They figure they can miss workouts. They assume it will be easy for them to make a comeback.

Of course, we know it's not that easy. A setback is like a little pothole in the road. It's not difficult to get out of the pothole if you work at it early enough. But the longer you stay in that hole—that emotional rut—the deeper the hole gets. You'll think it's that much harder to get going again. You'll eat poorly for a couple of meals, and then you'll decide to go ahead and eat badly the rest of the day. So you'll eat poorly for another day. Soon, your eating program is snowballing out of control. And it becomes really easy to quit.

So just as it's important to know how to start the North Program, it's equally important to know how to restart it.

Don't Get Down on Yourself

If you spend much time moping about a setback, you'll be doing more harm than good. It's hard to stay motivated when you're down on yourself.

If you know you're missing a workout, don't think you need to run an extra mile or lift weights for thirty extra minutes next time to catch up. That kind of thinking will inevitably make you hate exercise, because it's turning workouts into punishment. If you eat a group of cheat meals, don't make the mistake of thinking you need to cut way back on your meals for the next couple of days. Just resume the program at the next meal. Plan your menus very specifically for the day, write them down, study them. That way you won't deviate. And make sure your refrigerator is stocked with plenty of nonfat snack foods, such as carrots.

Your fitness depends on the everyday personal steps you take today and tomorrow. It does *not* depend on doing anything drastic. Here's a tip: Instead of visualizing yourself at your worst, visualize yourself at your best. If, in your mind, you hold an image of your body as you wish it to be, then you will want to stick with the program. A real key to this program is learning how to do "mind workouts," so that you forget about your imperfections and think only of the ways you are improving. Stay away from negative thoughts that can weigh you down and leave you drained and defeated.

If you talk to people who have been long-time adherents of the North Program, they will tell you that they actually stop worrying about tangible progress. They quit obsessing about losing another inch from their waists, because they know their bodies will keep getting better—as long as they stay on the program.

When You're Too Tired To Get Back into the Gym

This is going to sound crazy, but the best time for you to go to the gym is when you think you're absolutely too exhausted to work out.

You might very well be tired, but your feeling of fatigue is usually exaggerated. It is probably caused by that devilish part of your brain that wants you to be lazy.

Don't forget what we know about how the body works. Your body gets more energy from a workout than it does from a nap. The next time you're exhausted, try ten quick push-ups on your office floor. Or hold the back of your chair seat and lift your legs off the floor, bringing your knees to your waist (keep your back straight!).

Not much of a workout, you say? Perhaps not. But it will trigger a kind of muscle memory about how good it feels to work out. Your heart will pump more. You'll get that quick endorphin rush that comes from exercise. You may even want drop to the floor and do another set of push-ups. Or you might find yourself heading straight to the gym.

When I am feeling listless, I still go to the gym, but I do a very light workout. I don't try to kill myself. I'll walk on the treadmill or I'll do a light, fifteen-minute weight routine. Of course, usually after that fifteen minutes, I'm saying, "Hey, I feel pretty good. Let's go another fifteen minutes."

Try this fifteen-minute technique as an antidote for excuses. Remember, the longer you stay away from the gym, the harder it is to return.

No Time to Work Out?

Of course, lack of time is the number one excuse you can find to skip your workout.

First, I know you work hard and can't always control your schedule. On Monday, for example, you may have to work longer because it's the start of the week or you're on a big project and you're too busy to take an hour in the afternoon to get to the gym. On Tuesday, the same thing happens. It happens again Wednesday. By Thursday, you're getting worn down and you're still busy. That's when you start rationalizing. You'll say, "Well, I blew my workouts for that week. I'll wait until Monday and just start over."

I simply can't believe you can't find thirty minutes somewhere to work out. If you have time to eat, you have time to work out. Moreover, the basic benefit of exercise is that it gives you more vitality. You can concentrate more easily throughout the day and accomplish tasks more efficiently if you exercise. The right kind of exercise boosts your body's ability to take in oxygen and use it to make new energy.

If you don't exercise, you are saying that you're willing to accept possible obesity, bad blood circulation, shortened breath, and all of those minor aches and pains that you could get rid of simply by working out, those bothersome conditions that actually inhibit your productivity.

In other words, if you work out, you'll have more time on your hands—which means you'll always have time to work out.

Prepare for the Return of Bad Habits

Sometimes, when you feel your dedication starting to slip, you need a strategy to keep yourself from reverting to a bad habit. Be realistic about this. You can give yourself great speeches about staying pumped up all day long. But no speech is going to help you every time. Since you know you're inevitably going to fall into workout slumps, you also need to anticipate breaking them.

I know a guy who, when he feels the slump coming, sends a letter from his office to his house. The letter says, "Put down the mail and get on the bike." One of the things he uses as an excuse for not working out is grabbing his mail and sitting down in front of the television to read it. Soon he's got the remote control in his hand and he's watching the news. His letters to himself are a reminder of how easy it is to read *while riding his stationary cycle.*

One time, a woman who knew she was due for a slump handed me a CD she had just bought—a favorite musical group. "Don't let me have this until I work out three times this week," she said. I put the CD in a cabinet, and a week later—after her three workouts—she got it back. The point is, you need to devise whatever slump-buster works for you. Leave yourself messages on your answering machine, disconnect your TV, do whatever you have to do to prevent yourself from slipping off the program.

Run, Don't Walk, from Your Skeptics

One of the ways to avoid a setback is to start the program with someone who knows what you're going through. While you're the one who ultimately has to make the changes in your life, it doesn't hurt to talk about it with someone else. No doubt there's someone at the gym who knows exactly what you're thinking and feeling. Go to lunch with her! You'll both be ordering dishes without the extra fat, sharing stories, and urging each other on.

Another way to avoid a slump is to stay away from people who are unsupportive of your goals. At times, your friends can be your worst enemies. They'll say, "Do you really have to work out today? It's a holiday." "I know you're on a diet, but I made this pie especially for you." "Don't you think you're looking a little too thin?" It's even possible that they may be sabotaging you because they are jealous that you look so good. Or perhaps they resent your focusing more attention on yourself than on them. Whatever the reason, don't let naysayers interfere with your goals. Continue to make decisions based on your happiness, not on someone else's idea of what your happiness should be.

BUILDING YOUR OWN MOTIVATION

Before his death, my father and I reconciled. My brothers and I took care of him throughout the ordeal of cancer that took his life. It was then that I realized that despite the turmoil of my youth, my father did teach me one invaluable lesson. Unintentionally, he taught me persistence.

I realized that he had been deeply dedicated to his goals, even if they were goals that led him to endless failure and self-destruction. I became just as dedicated to my goals, though they differed wildly from his. I was not going to stop pursuing them, regardless of how many obstacles were put in front of me.

You, too, must embrace dedication. You must constantly keep up your momentum. This is a lesson for your life, as well as for your fitness program. While you may cheat at times, while you may suffer setbacks, while you may slow down, never, ever let yourself stop.

My father used to tell me over and over that he had finally turned the corner. He believed it, and I believed it. But then he would fail again. So when you start to feel really confident in your program, when you think you're really getting good, that's when you need to redouble your efforts to stay fit. Your dedication is not going to come out of thin air. Instead, you must master the art of self-motivation. The price of fitness is responsibility.

Of all the inspiring testimonials I have heard from people who've found a new lease on life in the North Program, one of the most inspiring came from a very down-on-his-luck, overweight man who lived in a boarding house. He wrote me and told me that he had plugged in an old AM radio and listened to my show as a form of entertainment. But over the months, after he kept listening to me say that people change their entire lives by taking care of themselves physically, he began to change. This man, who was close to homeless, had been eating mostly cheap processed and fried foods, foods high in salt and fat. But after listening to my show, he decided to buy a little hot plate, and he began buying oatmeal and rice, canned tuna and white chicken in water, and canned vegetables for fiber. He began eating five small meals a day, the price of which he said cost him less than one meal at a fast-food outlet. He didn't have proper shoes to jog with, so he started to walk, averaging thirty minutes five times a week. Within three months, his energy was up, his negative attitude was gone, and for the first time in a decade, he decided to pursue a goal that had eluded him. He wrote me that he had obtained a full-time job, found a place of his own to live, and lost thirty pounds.

If this man could find the motivation to adopt this program when he was barely keeping a roof over his head, then what excuse can the rest of us have?

FINAL THOUGHTS

I cannot tell you how excited I am that you've finished this book. Just by absorbing this program, you will almost certainly want to start following it. You will change your habits simply by becoming aware of what food does when it enters your body, by sensing the importance of the muscle tissues in your body, and by realizing the advantage of burning off a few extra calories through extra cardio activities.

There is nothing more satisfying to me than seeing people who realize they have found a program that actually works—that actually shapes their bodies. You know you can't feel truly successful if you do not feel good about your body. Now, you have that chance to feel good. Your physical changes will produce emotional changes, you'll feel better at work and at home, and you'll notice that people want to look at you. They'll want to be around you, because you exude rare energy and attractiveness.

I said it at the start of the book, and I'll say it again here: Any program that you can't do for the rest of your life is not worth doing for a single day. For as long as you live, you'll have the North Program. All you must do is keep believing in yourself.

I wish you the very best in your journey.

A p p e n d i x ■

MEALS FOR LIFE

■ If you are still a little worried that you will get bored eating the right kinds of foods, then worry no more. Here is a wide selection of tasty menus and meal plans for your eating pleasure.

The menus here—along with the sampling of very easy-to-cook dishes that I've already given you in Chapter Five—will give you more meals than you can ever hope to eat. Recipes for all dishes follow, as do recipes for a variety of specially prepared breakfasts.

W e e k   O n e

S u n d a y :
Chicken fajitas
Spanish rice (from mix)
Corn or pinto/black beans

M o n d a y :
Jamaican chicken feathers
Roasted potatoes
Carrots

T u e s d a y :
Chicken-baked steak
Mashed potatoes
Old-fashioned green beans

Wednesday:
Macaroni and cheese

Salad

Thursday:
Wild rice shrimp casserole

Steamed asparagus

Week Two

Monday:
Fake fried chicken

Mashed potatoes

Green beans/peas

Tuesday:
Beef with broccoli

Rice

Thai cucumber salad

Wednesday:
Vegetable lasagne

Salad

Thursday:
Shrimp scampi

Rice

Squash

Friday:
Stuffed turkey tenderloin

Sweet potatoes

Broccoli

Week Three

Monday:
Barbecued chicken

Rice

Squash

Tuesday:
Shrimp étouffée

Rice

French-cut green beans

Wednesday:
Mushroom risotto

Spinach or salad

Thursday:
Chicken and dumplings

Salad

.

Friday:
Boeuf bourguignonne

Roasted potatoes

Green beans or broccoli

Week Four

Monday:
Tamale pie

Corn or beans or salad

Tuesday:
Santa Fe chicken

Rice

Carrots

Wednesday:
Spinach ricotta dumplings

Pasta

Salad

Thursday:
Rice salad with chicken breast

Friday:
Pork with mustard sauce

Roasted potatoes

Green beans or broccoli

Week Five

Monday:
Buffalo chicken feathers

Rice

Corn casserole

Tuesday:
Chicken and ham jambalaya

Carrots

Wednesday:
Lemon shrimp fettuccine

Broccoli

Thursday:
Meatloaf

Mashed potato

Green beans or peas

Friday:
Carolina turkey

Wild rice

Corn

Week Six

Monday:
Chicken broccoli rice casserole

Salad

Tuesday:
Pizza

Salad

Wednesday:
Spaghetti

Spinach

Thursday:
Grilled lemon-lime chicken

Baked potato

Carrots

Friday:
Chicken cordon bleu

Rice

Green beans

This is only a small sampling of the various dishes you can try. Turn the page for a cornucopia of others.

RECIPES

Trim all visible fat off of all meats. Wash all vegetables. Cut the ends off of all vegetables with stalks, e.g., mushrooms, broccoli, celery, etc. Cut the stems off of carrots, eggplants, peppers, etc. Remove the ribs (the white part) and seeds from peppers. Peel the outer skin off onions and garlic unless otherwise indicated.

Granulated garlic and granulated onion are interchangeable with garlic powder and onion powder. The granules are less likely to cake and block the pouring holes, especially when one uses the jar over steaming foods.

It's recommended to rinse the tops of all cans before opening them.

All dairy products should be fat-free. All processed foods should be no added fat, e.g., tomato sauce without added oil.

Cover all cookie sheets or baking pans with foil when cooking meat (for easy clean-up without using fat).

Defat all broth.

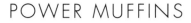 # POWER MUFFINS

MAKES ABOUT 12 MUFFINS

2 cups rolled oats

10 egg whites

2 Granny Smith apples, peeled and chopped

1 teaspoon cinnamon

½ teaspoon vanilla

3 packages Sweet 'n Low (not Equal*) or 3 teaspoons honey

1 teaspoon grated orange or lemon zest (optional)

½ cup raisins (optional)

Preheat oven to 375 degrees.

Combine all ingredients. Beat with an electric mixer about 2 minutes. Pour into nonstick muffin pans. Bake in preheated oven for 15 to 20 minutes. Store in zipper bags in refrigerator.

*Aspartame (Equal and Nutrasweet) products should not be used in cooking. These break down when heated, losing their sweetening power.

■ BREAKFAST ON THE RUN

This recipe is limited only by your imagination. Instead of rice you can use cooked hash browns, either cubed or shredded, and whatever strikes your fancy as flavoring ingredients.

3 cups cooked white or brown rice

1 cup grated fat-free cheese, divided in half (cheddar is best, can use Monterey jack)

4 ounces canned diced green chiles

2 ounces diced pimientos

⅓ cup skim milk

4 egg whites, beaten stiff

½ teaspoon ground cumin

½ teaspoon salt

½ teaspoon pepper

Preheat oven to 400 degrees.

Combine rice, ½ cup cheese, and all other ingredients except egg whites. Fold in beaten whites and divide batter among 12 muffin cups sprayed with nonstick cooking spray. Sprinkle with remaining cheese. Bake for about 15 minutes.

OPTIONAL INGREDIENTS

(The amount you use is up to your personal preference, a cup of chunky ingredients is a good starting point.) You can add or subtract according to your taste. For the herbs and spices start with ½ a teaspoon if they are dried, one tablespoon if they are fresh. This is a great way to use up leftover rice, vegetables or meat.

Chopped cooked mushrooms, bell pepper, onion, and ham or chicken

Chopped cooked spinach, Swiss cheese, mushrooms, and onion

Chopped cooked broccoli, onion, and chicken

Oats, chopped apples, and dried or fresh cinnamon

Diced jalapeño, chopped roasted red bell pepper, celery, and onion

Basil, oregano, chopped roasted bell pepper, and chopped artichoke hearts

Lemon pepper and Parmesan cheese

APPLE OAT MUFFINS

3½ cups rolled oats

¾ cup whole wheat flour

1 teaspoon apple or pumpkin pie spice

1½ teaspoons baking powder

½ teaspoon baking soda

¼ teaspoon salt

12 egg whites, slightly beaten

2 or 3 Granny Smith apples, peeled and diced

½ cup honey

Preheat oven to 350 degrees.

Mix the dry ingredients together. Make a well in the center and add the egg whites, apples, and honey. Stir just until the dry ingredients are moistened. Spoon into a muffin pan sprayed with nonstick spray. Bake in the preheated oven for 20 to 25 minutes.

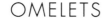 # OMELETS

The great thing about omelets is that you can put anything you like in them: meat, vegetables or even leftovers.

½ onion, diced

½ bell pepper, seeded and diced

½ cup sliced mushrooms

16 egg whites

Salt, pepper, granulated onion, and granulated garlic

Sauté the vegetables on medium heat. Cook until soft, set aside, and rinse skillet. While the vegetables are cooking, prepare the egg whites. Combine the seasonings to taste with the whites in a large bowl and whisk until foamy.

Reheat the skillet on low heat, pour in the egg whites, and sprinkle the vegetables evenly around the pan. Cover and set the timer for 7 to 10 minutes. (Watch your omelet the first few times you make it, so you'll know exactly how long it will take.) With a plastic spatula, loosen the edges and the underside of the omelet. Slide onto a plate and cut into 4 equal wedges.

■ BAKED POTATO SOUP

For the turkey garnish, buy very thin smoked turkey, either prepackaged or from the deli counter, separate the slices, and place on a paper towel. Microwave on high until crisp, starting at about a minute. The length of time the slices take to become crisp but not burned will vary between 30 seconds and 3 minutes, depending on the number of slices and the wattage of your microwave. Make sure you use plain smoked turkey; sugar, maple or honey cured will burn before it dehydrates completely.

> 1 cup mashed potatoes
>
> 2 cups defatted chicken broth
>
> 2 cups evaporated skim milk
>
> 2 baked potatoes, diced with the skin on
>
> ½ teaspoon granulated onion
>
> ¼ teaspoon granulated garlic
>
> 3 tablespoons Butter Buds
>
> ¼ cup chopped green onion

GARNISH:

> Grated nonfat Cheddar cheese
>
> Nonfat sour cream
>
> Smoked turkey slices, crisped and crumbled

Combine the mashed potatoes, broth, and skim milk in a saucepan. Heat over medium until simmering. Add the diced potatoes, seasonings, and green onion. Stir to mix well and reduce heat until soup is thick. Garnish with cheese, sour cream, crumbled turkey bacon, and additional green onion, if desired.

■ BLACK BEAN SOUP

I made this for a friend about ten years ago while we were sailing. To this day, he still talks about it. If you let the liquid evaporate until it's thick, it makes great nachos.

3 cloves garlic, peeled and minced

1 teaspoon cumin seeds

3 (15-ounce) cans black beans

1 bottle beer

1 onion, peeled and diced

1 jalapeño, sliced

¼ cup cilantro, leaves only coarsely chopped

Nonfat sour cream

Brown garlic and cumin seeds in a large saucepan. Add black beans, beer, onion, and jalapeño. Bring to a boil and reduce heat. Take out 1 to 1½ cups black beans and purée in a blender or food processor to thicken soup. Return purée to remaining soup and heat through, stirring to mix. Garnish with cilantro and sour cream.

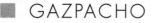 GAZPACHO

The perfect soup for summer.

> 2 cups V-8 regular or spicy, or tomato juice
>
> 2 large tomatoes, peeled, seeded, and chopped
>
> 1 green pepper, seeded and chopped
>
> 1 cucumber, seeded and chopped
>
> ½ onion, peeled and chopped
>
> 1 celery stalk, chopped
>
> 2 cloves garlic, peeled and minced
>
> 2 tablespoons red wine vinegar
>
> Salt, pepper, and hot pepper sauce to taste

Combine the ingredients and purée in a food processor or blender until smooth. Chill at least 1 hour before serving. Garnish with diced vegetables, croutons, or lime quarters, if desired.

■ SPICY SHRIMP SOUP

Substitute the zest of half a lemon if you can't find lemongrass. Fish sauce is the Thai and Vietnamese equivalent to soy sauce. It's very salty and smells very strongly of old fish, but as it cooks it mellows in both odor and flavor.

½ pound fresh shrimp

1 stalk fresh lemongrass, sliced

1 (8-ounce) can straw mushrooms, drained

1 to 2 tablespoons fish sauce

¼ cup fresh lime juice

2 fresh tomatoes, seeded and diced

2 tablespoons sliced green onion

1 tablespoon chopped cilantro

1 to 4 red chile peppers, seeded and chopped, or ½ teaspoon
    red chili paste

Peel and devein shrimp. Bring 1 quart of water to a boil and add lemongrass and straw mushrooms. Reduce heat to medium-low. Add shrimp; cook about 3 minutes. Add fish sauce, lime juice, and tomatoes; stir. Add green onions, cilantro, and red chile peppers. Stir well, remove from heat and serve.

■ ASPARAGUS GUACAMOLE

Try this with fat-free sour cream instead of mayonnaise. Canned asparagus is the key; fresh and frozen just don't have the right texture (mush).

1 (14-ounce) can asparagus, drained

1 cup tomato, diced and seeded (about 1 large tomato)

⅓ cup peeled, diced onion

2 tablespoons minced cilantro

2 tablespoons fat-free mayonnaise or Miracle Whip

1 tablespoon freshly squeezed lime juice

6 drops red pepper sauce

1 clove garlic, peeled and minced

¼ cup picante sauce, drained of excess liquid

Purée the asparagus in the food processor until smooth. Combine with all other ingredients, cover, and refrigerate at least 1 hour. Serve with baked corn tortilla chips.

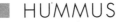 # HUMMUS

This dip is traditionally high in fat, since tahini (sesame seed paste) and olive oil are ingredients usually found in hummus. This variation is different, but still tastes Middle Eastern.

2 cans garbanzo beans (chick-peas), drained, liquid reserved

¼ to ½ cup fresh lemon juice

1 teaspoon garlic powder or 4 cloves garlic, crushed

½ teaspoon paprika

1 teaspoon ground cumin

Salt to taste

In a food processor or blender, purée the garbanzo beans with all the seasonings until smooth. Add the reserved liquid if necessary to achieve the desired consistency. Sprinkle a little paprika and ground cumin on top before serving, if you like.

BUFFALO CHICKEN FEATHERS

¼ cup (or more) cayenne pepper sauce (Louisiana Red Hot
    Sauce, available in supermarkets)
1 package Butter Buds
3 pounds chicken tenders
1 cup flour
1 teaspoon onion powder
Chicken broth in a spray bottle
Celery and carrot sticks

Preheat oven to 425 degrees.

Combine hot sauce, butter buds, and chicken tenders and marinate for at least 1 hour. Put flour and onion powder in a large plastic zip bag. Add marinated chicken and shake until coated. Place the tenders on a rack over a roasting pan, spray with defatted chicken broth, and bake until they are brown, 15 to 20 minutes, turning them after 10 minutes or so. Serve with celery and carrot sticks.

Marinade Variation

TANGY CHINESE FEATHERS

¾ cup dark soy sauce
1 tablespoon (or more) grated fresh gingerroot
2 garlic cloves, peeled and finely minced
⅓ cup brown sugar
1 tablespoon Chinese mustard

Combine marinade ingredients in a large plastic zip bag, add about 3 pounds of chicken tenders and marinate at least one hour. For crispy feathers, follow the instructions above. For a variation, cook without dredging in flour.

JAMAICAN CHICKEN FEATHERS

⅓ cup dark rum

⅓ cup dark soy sauce

1 egg white, slightly beaten

2 tablespoons freshly grated fresh gingerroot (not necessary to peel)

2 garlic cloves, peeled and finely minced

Combine marinade ingredients in a large plastic zip bag. Add about 3 pounds of chicken tenders. Close and marinate at least 1 hour. Follow cooking instructions for buffalo chicken feathers.

■ PIZZA PIZZA PIZZA

Begin with a fat-free crust. You can make it using a pizza dough recipe or buy one at the store. Be creative. If you can't find a crust specifically made for pizza, try something like pita bread. You can make your own tomato sauce or buy one of the fat-free sauces that comes in a jar and spice it up with a little extra basil, oregano, crushed red pepper, and garlic. You can also be imagi--native with the toppings.

BARBECUE PIZZA

Pour barbecue sauce on top of your crust (use a cornmeal-based crust if you wish). Top with:

*Grated fat-free Cheddar cheese (Lifetime brand if you can
    find it)*
Sliced grilled chicken
Thinly sliced or chopped and peeled red onion
Jalapeños (optional)

Broil or bake at 400 degrees for about 8 minutes, or until the cheese melts.

MEXICAN PIZZA

Spread fat-free "refried" beans on top of your crust (again, cornmeal if you like). Sprinkle with:

Seasoned ground meat (lean beef, chicken, or turkey); Lawry's
    makes a great taco meat seasoning mix
Grated fat free Cheddar or Monterey Jack cheese
Chopped lettuce
Chopped tomatoes
Diced Onion
Fat-free sour cream and salsa or picante sauce

Broil or bake as above.

ORIENTAL PIZZA

Spread plum or hoisin sauce on top of your crust. Top with:

Shrimp or shredded chicken (a nice touch is to marinate it in a
    mixture of soy, ginger, and garlic)
Shredded raw cabbage
Shredded carrots
Chopped green onion

Bake or broil until heated through.

CLASSIC VEGETABLE PIZZA

Spread tomato sauce on top of your crust. Top with:

Fat-free mozzarella cheese, grated
Sliced mushrooms
Diced green pepper
Diced onion

Bake or broil until cheese melts.

BREAKFAST PIZZA

Spread softly scrambled egg whites on top of your crust (whole wheat would be a good choice). Top with:

Smoked turkey breast "bacon"
Grated fat-free Cheddar cheese
Diced green onion

Bake or broil as above.

MIDDLE EASTERN PIZZA

Spread fat-free hummus on top of your crust. Top with:

Diced tomatoes
Chopped parsley
Ground cumin

Bake or broil until heated through.

■ CHICKEN BROCCOLI RICE CASSEROLE

SERVES 4

This is a great way to use up leftover chicken or rice. If you don't like broccoli, you can always substitute a vegetable you prefer, such as turnip, collard greens, mustard, or spinach. All you need is a salad to make this a complete meal.

One of the local morning show hosts loves this recipe. When it was demonstrated on TV one morning, we received more than 300 requests for the recipe.

1 pound boneless, skinless chicken breasts, trimmed of fat, cut in chunks

Flour, salt, pepper, and garlic powder for dredging

1 large onion, peeled and chopped

4 cloves garlic, peeled and minced

Defatted chicken broth for sautéing

1 can 99 percent fat-free cream of mushroom soup

½ pound fresh mushrooms, sliced, or 1 jar sliced mushrooms

Salt, pepper, and garlic powder

8 ounces nonfat cheese (Cheddar or American), grated, or 1 envelope dehydrated cheese from a packaged macaroni and cheese mix

1 pound broccoli florets, fresh or defrosted frozen

5 cups cooked rice

Preheat oven to 350 degrees.

Dredge the chicken chunks in the flour/seasoning mixture. Brown the chicken in a large nonstick skillet. Set aside. Brown the onion and garlic in a small amount of broth, using the same skillet that has the chicken "drippings." When the onion has softened, add the cream of mushroom soup and mushrooms, and season with salt, pepper and garlic powder to taste. Add the nonfat cheese and mix well until the sauce is a uniform color. Add fresh broccoli florets to the sauce and cook about 5 minutes. Mix the chicken, rice, and sauce together. Put in an ovenproof casserole and bake in a preheated 350-degree oven until bubbly, about 30 to 40 minutes.

■ CHICKEN AND DUMPLINGS

1 pound boneless, skinless chicken breasts, trimmed of fat,
  chopped in bite-size pieces

½ cup whole wheat or all-purpose flour

Chicken broth for sautéing and baking

½ cup dry white wine

1 large onion, peeled and chopped

4 cloves garlic, peeled and minced

4 carrots, sliced in ½-inch rounds

4 medium potatoes, cut into chunks

2 celery stalks, chopped

1 pound fresh mushrooms, sliced

1 tablespoon chopped fresh rosemary, or 1 teaspoon dry

½ teaspoon pepper

½ teaspoon garlic powder

½ teaspoon salt

½ teaspoon onion powder

1 teaspoon Italian seasoning

Preheat oven to 350 degrees.

Dredge the chicken in the flour seasoned with next five in-gredients. (Save the excess flour for the dumplings.) Heat a non-stick skillet on medium heat, pour in a little broth, and let brown and evaporate. Brown small amounts of the floured chicken in the pan, pouring in a little broth if needed to loosen. Set aside as the chicken is browned. Add wine, onion, and garlic to skillet and cook on medium for a couple of minutes. Add the carrots and cook a few minutes longer, stirring often. Add the potatoes and cook about 5 minutes. Pour the contents of the skillet into a large glass Pyrex dish. Add the celery, mushrooms, rosemary, and browned chicken. Adjust the seasonings, add more salt, pepper, onion powder or garlic powder as needed. Stir to mix well. Pour in enough chicken broth to cover. Mix up dumpling mixture and drop by spoonfuls onto the chicken mixture. Cover with foil and bake in the preheated oven for about 40 minutes.

An alternate method of cooking, is on top of the stove. Begin by browning your chicken in a large saucepan or Dutch oven. Follow the instructions as above, but instead of pouring into a Pyrex, continue cooking on top of the stove. Bring mixture to a boil, reduce heat to a simmer and cook for about 20 minutes before adding the dumpling mixture. Drop by spoonfuls into the simmering liquid and cover immediately. Do not remove cover until dumplings are done.

DUMPLINGS:

1 cup flour

2 teaspoons baking powder

½ teaspoon salt

Your choice of garlic powder, crushed rosemary, thyme, or dill to taste

Up to ½ cup water or skim milk

Mix dry ingredients together. Stir the milk slowly into the dry mixture. Keep batter "stiff."

■ CHICKEN CORDON BLEU

This can be changed to saltimbocca just by sprinkling a little sage on the inside of the chicken breasts.

4 boneless, skinless breasts

4 slices nonfat Swiss cheese

4 slices smoked turkey or lean ham

½ cup nonfat bread crumbs

1 egg white

¼ cup skim milk

Salt, pepper, onion powder, and garlic powder

Chicken broth in a spray bottle

Preheat oven to 350 degrees.

Pound the breasts until they are tender and somewhat flattened. Place a slice of cheese and one of ham on one side of each pounded breast. Fold the other side over, press the edges together to seal, and coat the chicken in bread crumbs. In a small bowl, mix the milk, egg white, and seasonings to taste. Dip the breaded chicken in the egg wash and dip again in the bread crumbs. Place the chicken on a foil-covered cookie sheet and spray with broth. Bake for 20 minutes.

QUICK FAJITAS

SERVES 4

Liquid Fajita Marinade (recipe follows)
4 boneless, skinless chicken breasts, trimmed of fat, or 1 pound
*   of lean beef*
Defatted chicken broth
2 onions, peeled and sliced
2 bell peppers, green or red, sliced in strips
2 limes
Fat-free tortillas

Marinate chicken. Grill, broil, or pan-sauté chicken breasts in small amount of chicken broth. Heat skillet on high, let it get hot, add about 2 tablespoons chicken broth, and let it brown. Add onions and green peppers and let the edges of the onions brown. Add broth as needed, or a squeeze of lime juice. Stir occasionally. Cook until tender. Thinly slice the chicken and put a few strips inside a fat-free flour tortilla with some of the pepper mixture on top. Roll up and serve with pico de gallo, Spanish rice, and beans.

HOMEMADE FAJITA MARINADE

2 teaspoons liquid smoke
¼ cup water
4 teaspoons soy sauce
1 teaspoon A-1 sauce
3 teaspoons sugar
Juice of 1 lime

Combine all ingredients and mix well. Marinate chicken or beef in refrigerator overnight if possible, or for at least 2 hours.

■ FAKE FRIED CHICKEN

Empty refillable trigger spray bottles are found in the pharmacy section of most grocery stores. Fill them with the appropriate de-fatted broth and refrigerate for up to 3 days. If you boil the broth every three days, it will keep much longer.

You can dredge your chicken in a variety of batters and crumbs. Try nonfat or 1 percent buttermilk or nonfat yogurt. You can use a combination of flour and breadcrumbs or toasted oatmeal that you've ground in the food processor. You can also add cornmeal. (Fake fried fish is best with a combination of flour and cornmeal.) The most important step for a great-tasting crust using flour, cornmeal, or oatmeal is to make sure you wet your coating thoroughly with broth. No dry spots should remain. The moisture makes it cook properly so it doesn't taste raw.

4 boneless, skinless chicken breasts, trimmed of fat

1 cup fine dry bread crumbs

1 teaspoon garlic powder

1 teaspoon Italian herb seasoning or your favorite blend

Salt and pepper

1 egg white

½ cup skim milk

Defatted chicken broth in a spray bottle

Preheat oven to 350 degrees.

Trim all visible fat from chicken. Wash and pat dry. Combine all dry ingredients in a gallon size plastic zip bag. Add chicken and shake. Beat egg white and milk together in bowl. Dip breaded chicken in egg mixture. Put chicken back in plastic bag and shake again. Place chicken on foil-covered cookie sheet. Mist with chicken broth until moist and bake for 20 to 30 minutes in the preheated oven. The traditional accompaniments are mashed potatoes and either peas or green beans.

GRILLED LEMON-LIME CHICKEN

Grated zest (about 2 teaspoons) and juice (about ¾ cup) of 2
  lemons
Grated zest (about 2½ teaspoons) and juice (about ¾ cup) of 3
  limes
1½ tablespoons sugar
1 teaspoon finely chopped garlic
¼ teaspoon cayenne pepper
Salt and pepper
8 boneless, skinless chicken breasts

In a saucepan whisk together the zests, juices, sugar, garlic, cayenne, and salt and pepper to taste. Bring the mixture to a boil, reduce the heat, and simmer, stirring, for 5 minutes, or until the sugar is dissolved. Let cool. In a large plastic zipper bag place the chicken, pricked in several places with a fork, and pour in the marinade. Seal and shake, then let the chicken marinate in the refrigerator, turning it once, for 1 to 3 hours. Transfer the chicken with tongs to a grill set about 6 inches over glowing coals, or to a ridged grill pan set over moderately high heat, and grill it, basting it with the marinade for the first 10 minutes (discard any remaining marinade). Turn the chicken over and grill it for 10 minutes more, or until it is cooked through.

■ CHICKEN AND HAM JAMBALAYA

SERVES 4

You can really spice this up either by using a Cajun spice mixture or as much Tabasco as your taste buds can take.

2 to 3 cups defatted chicken broth

1 pound boneless, skinless chicken breasts, trimmed of fat, cut into bite-size pieces

½ pound lean ham, cut into bite-size pieces

3 cloves garlic, peeled and minced

1 medium onion, peeled and minced

3 medium tomatoes, peeled, seeded, and chopped

1 medium bell pepper, seeded and diced

2 stalks celery, diced

½ teaspoon crushed oregano

¼ teaspoon cayenne pepper

½ teaspoon crushed thyme

1 bunch green onions, chopped (greens too)

4 cups cooked rice

Salt and pepper

Heat a skillet on high, add a couple of tablespoons of the broth, and let brown. Add chicken, ham, and garlic. Brown, stirring constantly, about 10 minutes. Add onion, tomatoes, bell pepper, and celery. Cook until onion is soft. Add 2 cups of remaining broth and the oregano, pepper, and thyme. Cover and simmer about 15 minutes, stirring often. Add the green onions and rice. Stir to mix well. Remove from heat, cover, and let stand 5 to 10 minutes before serving, adding a bit more broth if the mixture seems too dry.

■ RICE SALAD

This recipe is a great way to use leftovers. Other things you can add are marinated artichokes, capers, or a few olives. Instead of sautéing the mushrooms, quite often I marinate them in vinaigrette for a few hours.

I'm not sure why nonfat mayo has to be sweet, but to "tart" it up a bit, I add 1 tablespoon of wine vinegar or lemon juice, ¼ teaspoon dry mustard, and a sprinkle of paprika.

8 ounces fresh mushrooms, sliced

Chicken broth for sautéing

1 cup defrosted frozen corn

2 cups cold cooked rice

4 cooked, boneless, skinless chicken breasts, diced

½ green bell pepper, seeded and diced

1 medium onion, peeled and diced

1 can Le Sueur® peas, drained, or 1 cup fresh or defrosted
   frozen tiny peas

1 small jar diced pimientos, or diced roasted red peppers

1 cup nonfat mayonnaise

½ cup nonfat vinaigrette (recipe follows)

½ teaspoon each garlic and onion powder

Salt and pepper

2 ripe tomatoes, seeded, and diced

Sauté mushrooms in chicken broth until soft and slightly brown around the edges. Remove from heat and place in a large bowl. Warm corn in the same pan. Drain and combine with mushrooms. Add rice, chicken, green pepper, onion, peas, pimiento, mayonnaise, and vinaigrette. Add seasonings, adjusting to taste. Cover with plastic wrap and refrigerate overnight. Just before serving, add tomatoes. Toss to mix well. This is a great summer entrée.

VINAIGRETTE

¼ to ⅓ cup red wine vinegar

1 teaspoon Italian herb seasoning, crushed

¼ cup skim milk

1 to 2 teaspoons Dijon mustard

Salt, pepper, garlic, and onion powder

SANTA FE CHICKEN

SERVES 4

⅓ cup all purpose flour

1 teaspoon chili powder

½ teaspoon granulated garlic

½ teaspoon onion powder

½ teaspoon paprika

¼ teaspoon red pepper

½ teaspoon cumin

½ teaspoon salt

4 boneless, skinless chicken breasts

½ cup defatted chicken broth in a spray bottle

Preheat oven to 350 degrees.

Combine all dry ingredients in a plastic zip bag. Add the chicken breasts and shake to coat well. Place chicken on a foil-covered baking sheet and spray with chicken broth until no dry spots remain. Bake for 20 minutes.

■ CAROLINA TURKEY

This has been adapted from a *Dallas Morning News* recipe. Serve it with either rice or potatoes. If you slice your turkey into bite-size strips, you can toss it all together with pasta.

4 turkey breast steaks
Salt and freshly ground pepper
½ cup flour
1 can defatted chicken broth
2 tablespoons minced shallots
2 tablespoons red wine vinegar
1 cup skinned, seeded, diced tomatoes
1 pound frozen or fresh corn
¼ cup evaporated skim milk
1 teaspoon Dijon-style mustard
Salt and pepper
¼ cup coarsely chopped basil leaves

Pound the turkey breasts with a cleaver or meat tenderizer until about ⅛ thick. Sprinkle both sides with salt and pepper to taste and dredge them in flour, shaking off the excess. Heat a small amount of chicken broth in a large skillet. When it is hot, add the meat and brown lightly on both sides, continuing to cook about 5 minutes or until done. Add a few tablespoons of broth as needed to keep from burning. Transfer to a serving platter, cover, and keep warm. Add shallots to skillet and cook briefly, stirring. Add vinegar and simmer briefly. Add tomatoes, corn, and ⅓ cup chicken broth. Bring to a boil, stir, and cook for about 2 minutes. Add the milk and mustard and stir to blend. Add salt and pepper to taste and cook about 30 seconds. Add the basil and pour sauce over the meat. Serve immediately.

■ STUFFED TURKEY TENDERLOIN

You can make some very simple glazes to keep your turkey moist. Combine honey with bourbon or brandy, or use a frozen concentrated fruit juice like apple or orange. Maple syrup or brown sugar can also be used as the sweetener.

¼ cup dried cranberries

2 tablespoons bourbon or brandy

1 pound turkey tenderloin, tendon removed

Poultry seasoning

Onion powder

Garlic powder

½ Granny Smith apple, peeled, cored, and finely chopped

1 cup whole wheat bread crumbs

⅛ teaspoon crushed sage

2 egg whites, slightly beaten

1 tablespoon skim milk or water

Preheat oven to 400 degrees.

Soak the cranberries in the bourbon. Pound the tenderloin until thin, but not until it splits. Remove the thick white tendon. Sprinkle with poultry seasoning and onion and garlic powder. Combine the soaked cranberries with the finely chopped apple, bread crumbs, sage, egg whites, and milk. Mix well. Spread the stuffing on the turkey almost to the edges. Roll up and place seam side down in a shallow baking dish. Bake in the preheated oven for 50 to 60 minutes, brushing on glaze (recipe follows) from time to time.

Notes: It's very important to preheat your oven for this recipe. You may add grated orange peel to the stuffing or crumble rosemary on top. Slice the turkey just before serving to keep it from drying out.

GLAZE

½ cup unsweetened apple cider

2 tablespoons honey

⅛ teaspoon thyme

1 clove garlic, peeled and minced

Mix all the ingredients and brush on the turkey.

LEMON SHRIMP FETTUCCINE

SERVES 4

1 pound shrimp, peeled and deveined

Lemon pepper to taste

1 cup evaporated skim milk

1 package Butter Buds

2 tablespoons freshly squeezed lemon juice

8 teaspoons grated lemon peel (about 4 lemons)

1 pound fettuccine

Marinate shrimp in white wine or lemon juice. Sprinkle with lemon pepper and set aside. Heat a skillet on medium. Pour in the evaporated skim milk and Butter Buds. Mix thoroughly and heat until simmering, stirring occasionally. Add lemon juice and zest. Continue stirring as sauce thickens. Cook about 5 to 10 minutes. In a separate skillet, cook the shrimp just until done. Cook the fettuccine until it is al dente. Drain very well. Toss the pasta with sauce and shrimp. Serve immediately.

Variations

You can add artichoke hearts, capers, or asparagus tips.

■ SHRIMP ÉTOUFFÉE

2 tablespoons flour

1 medium onion, peeled and chopped

1 bell pepper, seeded and chopped

4 stalks celery, chopped

2 cloves garlic, peeled and minced

1 cup defatted chicken broth

1 pound shrimp, shelled and deveined

½ teaspoon hot pepper sauce

1 teaspoon salt

⅛ teaspoon freshly ground black pepper

⅛ teaspoon ground red pepper

½ cup chopped parsley

3 to 4 cups hot cooked rice

In a large cast-iron skillet, heat flour until medium-brown. Add the onion, bell pepper, celery, garlic, and a small amount of broth and cook until vegetables have softened. Stir in remaining broth, and seasonings. Simmer uncovered for 10 minutes. Add the shrimp and simmer just until shrimp is cooked, about 5 minutes. Serve over hot rice.

■ SHRIMP SCAMPI

SERVES 4

MARINADE

3 tablespoons dry vermouth
2 tablespoons minced Italian parsley
1 teaspoon olive oil
½ teaspoon salt
Pinch of pepper

1 pound shrimp, shelled and deveined
1 cup defatted chicken broth
10 garlic cloves, minced
1 cup dry white wine
1 package Butter Buds
Parsley sprigs and lemon slices for garnish

Mix marinade ingredients in a shallow glass bowl and marinate the shrimp for 2 or 3 hours.

Pour a couple of teaspoons of broth in a skillet. After the broth evaporates and browns, add the garlic and brown, adding broth as needed to keep from burning. Add the marinated shrimp and cook on medium heat until the shrimp curls. Add the white wine and Butter Buds, stir until the sauce thickens. Remove from heat and serve on a bed of buttered rice.

BUTTERED RICE

4 cups defatted chicken broth
2 cups raw white rice
1 onion, peeled and minced
½ package Butter Buds

Bring the broth, rice, and onion to a boil in a medium saucepan. Cover and reduce heat. Cook for 20 minutes. Remove from heat and stir in Butter Buds.

WILD RICE SHRIMP CASSEROLE

Try this with chicken or turkey chunks, if you don't like shrimp. You can use chopped fresh asparagus instead of artichokes. Garnish with cilantro or lemon slices. This has been adapted from a *Dallas Morning News* recipe.

1 pound raw shrimp, shelled and deveined

½ cup white wine

1 teaspoon lemon pepper

2 packages Uncle Ben's wild and long grain rice

½ teaspoon crushed red pepper flakes

1 can artichoke hearts, drained and cut in bite-size pieces

8 ounces nonfat sour cream

Marinate the shrimp in the wine and lemon pepper for about 30 minutes. Bring 3½ cups water to a boil, pour in the rice, seasoning packages, and red pepper. Stir to mix, cover, and simmer 10 minutes. Add the shrimp, cover again, and simmer 10 minutes longer, or until both the shrimp and the rice are cooked. Remove from heat and stir in the artichokes and sour cream.

■ BEEF WITH BROCCOLI

1 pound lean round steak, slightly frozen

1 teaspoon rice wine vinegar or dry sherry

1 tablespoon soy sauce, plus a bit for simmering

1 teaspoon sesame oil (optional)

1 teaspoon cornstarch

1 teaspoon peeled and minced fresh gingerroot

8 cloves garlic, peeled and minced

1 pound fresh broccoli

Chicken or beef broth for sautéing

Thinly slice the beef. Combine the vinegar or sherry, 1 table-spoon of the soy, sesame oil, cornstarch, ginger, and 4 cloves of minced garlic. Add to the sliced beef and mix to coat. Rinse and trim the broccoli and cut the florets into bite-size pieces; slice the stems diagonally. Heat a little oil or broth in a skillet on medium heat. When skillet is hot, add the remaining garlic and brown. Add the beef and stir-fry until desired doneness is reached. Remove from pan. Turn heat up to high and stir-fry the broccoli stems. Add the florets. Stir-fry for 1 minute. Add a little broth, soy sauce, and ¼ cup water. Reduce heat to medium, cover, and simmer. Add beef after about 10 minutes and heat through for a few minutes. Serve over rice.

APPENDIX: RECIPES *227* ■

■ BOEUF BOURGUIGNONNE

This is very rich-tasting (no one will guess it is low in fat), perfect for company on a cold winter evening. Since it takes a bit of time to prepare, I recommend making extra; it is worth every mouthful and minute, and keeps well in the refrigerator for a few days.

4 slices of lean Canadian bacon, in strips

3 tablespoons flour

1 teaspoon onion powder

Salt and pepper

1½ pounds round steak, sliced in 2-inch strips

1 medium onion, peeled and chopped

4 cloves garlic, peeled and minced

2 cups defatted beef broth

1½ cups Burgundy

1 tablespoon tomato paste

1 teaspoon bouquet garni, crushed, or 1 bouquet garni

12 to 16 pearl onions

1 cup defatted chicken broth

8 ounces fresh mushrooms, sliced

Preheat oven to 325 degrees.

Brown the Canadian bacon in a large skillet. Remove and set aside. Mix the flour, onion powder, salt, and pepper in a large plastic zip bag. Put the steak slices in, seal, and shake. Brown the beef, a small amount at a time, in a dry skillet. Be careful not to add too much meat at one time, or it won't brown. As each batch is browned, set aside with the Canadian bacon in a large oven-proof casserole. When the beef is finished, brown the chopped onion and the garlic in the same skillet. Add the beef broth, Burgundy, and tomato paste. Bring to a boil and pour over the beef. Add the bouquet garni and cover the casserole. Bake, covered, for 3 to 4 hours. While the beef is cooking, cook the pearl onions until tender. Put 2 tablespoons of chicken broth in a large skillet. Heat on medium-high until almost evaporated, then add the cooked pearl onions and the mushrooms and brown, adding broth as needed. When the beef is tender, remove from the oven and remove the bouquet garni if you used a sachet. Add the onions and mushrooms, stirring to mix well. Serve over "buttered" no-yolk egg noodles. (Toss the hot cooked noodles with a package of Butter Buds.)

 # CHICKEN-BAKED STEAK

SERVES 6 TO 8 (COUNT ¼ TO ⅓ POUND
MEAT PER SERVING)

You'd better make plenty; this is sure to disappear quickly.

2-pound eye of round roast, trimmed of all fat

1 cup flour

1½ teaspoons onion powder

1½ teaspoons granulated garlic

¼ teaspoon salt

¼ teaspoon pepper

3 egg whites

⅔ cup skim milk

Salt and pepper

1 cup defatted beef broth

Preheat oven to 500 degrees.

Cut the roast in ½-inch-thick slices. Pound to tenderize until each is about ¼ inch thick. In a large plastic zip bag or a pie pan, combine flour, 1 teaspoon onion powder, granulated garlic, salt, and pepper. Mix well. In a small bowl combine the egg whites, skim milk, remaining ½ teaspoon onion powder, garlic powder and additional salt and pepper. One piece at a time, dredge the meat in the flour mixture. Dip in the milk mixture. Dredge again in the seasoned flour. Place on a foil-covered cookie sheet. Pour the beef broth in a clean sprayer and spray the steaks until completely covered with broth. Place the cookie sheet in the oven and bake the meat slices for 20 minutes, or until brown and crispy. Serve immediately.

■ MOST REQUESTED MEATLOAF

1½ pounds ground beef or turkey or combination, at least 90
    percent lean

½ cup tomato sauce, V-8 juice, or tomato soup

1 medium onion, peeled and chopped

1 bell pepper, seeded and chopped

2 egg whites

¾ cup quick or old-fashioned rolled oats

1 package onion soup mix

1 teaspoon garlic powder

Couple of shakes Worcestershire sauce

Salt and pepper

1 can Zesty tomato soup (Italian tomato basil soup)

Preheat oven to 350 degrees.

Place meat in a large bowl. Combine all the other ingredients except zesty tomato soup in a medium bowl and mix thoroughly. Make a well in the meat and put the contents of the medium bowl in the well. Mix well. Place a cooling rack in the middle of a foil-lined roasting pan. After putting meat mixture in a loaf pan to shape, turn it out on the rack. Bake for 45 minutes. Top with zesty tomato soup and continue baking another ½ hour. Let stand 10 minutes before slicing.

Note: For an even leaner meatloaf, use less beef and more ground turkey breast, or more oatmeal, onion, and egg whites, or add chopped mushrooms or grated carrots. If you don't like tomato soup, try topping your meatloaf with barbecue sauce.

■ SPAGHETTI SAUCE

1 pound ground beef, 90 percent lean

1 (15-ounce) can tomato sauce

½ cup chopped onion

1 toaspoon minced garlic

½ cup chopped green pepper

2 tablespoons tomato paste

½ teaspoon fennel

½ cup dry white or red wine

1 teaspoon Italian herb seasoning

Pinch crushed red pepper

Brown ground meat, place in colander, rinse in hot water, and drain. In a clean saucepan, brown onion, garlic, and green pepper. Add meat and all other ingredients, and 1 cup of water. Simmer 20 minutes.

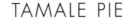 TAMALE PIE

½ cup yellow cornmeal

½ cup chicken broth, plus more for browning onion

⅓ cup nonfat yogurt

½ teaspoon salt

1 medium onion, peeled and finely chopped

2 cloves garlic, minced

1 pound ground beef (see Notes)

1 can crushed tomatoes or ½ cup picante sauce

1 tablespoon chili powder

½ teaspoon oregano, crumbled

½ teaspoon ground cumin

⅛ teaspoon pepper

1 cup defrosted frozen corn

½ cup nonfat Cheddar cheese, grated or shredded

4 sprigs cilantro

Preheat oven to 350 degrees.

Combine cornmeal, ½ cup broth, yogurt, and ¼ teaspoon salt in a bowl, stir well, and set aside. Sauté onion in a little broth; add garlic. In another pan, brown the ground beef. When done, place in colander and rinse with hot water. Add meat to onion mixture and stir the crushed tomatoes or picante sauce and corn. Add seasonings and stir. Pour the beef into a baking dish, then spread the cornmeal mixture on top. Sprinkle with the cheese. Bake for 20 minutes or until bubbly. Garnish with cilantro sprigs. Serve with a green salad topped with pico de gallo.

Notes: You can also use skinless, boneless chicken breasts. Slice in strips against the grain and simmer in broth until meat becomes tender enough to shred. Shred the meat and add to onion mixture. Proceed with recipe. This can easily be made into a vegetarian dish by substituting pinto or black beans for the meat.

◼ PORK WITH MUSTARD SAUCE

SERVES 6

1½ to 2 pounds pork tenderloin, trimmed of fat

½ cup plus 2 tablespoons defatted chicken broth

1 teaspoon thyme

1 medium onion, peeled and minced

8 cloves garlic, minced

1 bay leaf

1 tablespoon balsamic or red wine vinegar

1 tablespoon Dijon mustard

1 tablespoon Butter Buds

3 cornichons, chopped (optional)

Slice the tenderloin into ½-inch-thick slices. Heat 2 tablespoons of broth in a skillet. Brown pork on one side (about 5 minutes). Turn, add thyme and bay leaf. Cook until pork is cooked through (abut 5 minutes). Remove pork and keep warm. Add onion and garlic to skillet and brown. Add bay leaf, remaining broth, and vinegar, stir well, and reduce. Add mustard, Butter Buds, cornichons, and any liquid from meat. Stir and bring to a simmer. Remove the bay leaf. Pour sauce over meat and serve.

◼ MUSHROOM RISOTTO

4-plus cups defatted chicken broth

1 onion, peeled and thinly sliced

8 ounces bottled sliced mushrooms, or ¼ cup chopped dried
    porcini or morel mushrooms

¾ cup sauterne or favorite white wine

2 cups arborio or brown short-grain rice

Grated Parmesan-Reggiano cheese (optional)

Heat a couple of tablespoons of the chicken broth in a large, heavy skillet. Add the onion and cook until transparent. Drain the mushrooms if using canned, or soak if using dried. Add to the onion and mix well. Add the wine and stir. Simmer until the pan is almost dry. Add the rice and cook over low heat, stirring constantly, for about 5 minutes. Add 1 cup of broth and stir to mix well. Cook until almost all of the broth has been absorbed, stirring almost constantly. Continue adding broth 1 cup at a time, stirring constantly until the broth is almost completely absorbed each time. Serve as a main or side dish.

Quick method: After the first cup of broth has been absorbed, add the remaining broth, stir, and cover. Simmer, stirring frequently, about 25 minutes for arborio or 45 minutes for brown rice. Remove from heat. Add cheese if desired.

■ SPINACH RICOTTA DUMPLINGS

SERVES 4

This seems like a lot of spinach, but it's not a misprint.

1½ pounds frozen spinach, defrosted and dried

1 onion, peeled and minced

½ cup nonfat ricotta cheese, or ½ cup puréed nonfat cottage
    cheese

1 tablespoon minced garlic

½ teaspoon oregano

2 chicken bouillon cubes, crushed

¾ cup bread crumbs

3 egg whites

Black pepper

Nutmeg

Preheat oven to 325 degrees.

Combine all ingredients; mix well. Chill to firm up. Roll the mixture into balls about 1 to 1½ inches in diameter. Place the dumplings in a shallow baking dish. Place in the oven with a pan of hot water on the lower shelf to prevent the dumplings from drying out. Bake 10 to 15 minutes, or until lightly golden. Serve with a marinara sauce. This mixture can also be used as a stuffing for pasta shells.

■ VEGETABLE LASAGNE

8 ounces lasagna noodles

3 medium tomatoes, chopped

8 ounces tomato sauce

6 ounces tomato paste

1 medium green pepper, seeded and chopped

2 medium onions, peeled and chopped

½ teaspoon rosemary

½ teaspoon oregano

½ teaspoon thyme

½ teaspoon basil

8 ounces fresh mushrooms, sliced

1 medium bunch of broccoli, broken into florets

1 medium red (or green) pepper, seeded and chopped

1 large zucchini, sliced

4 teaspoons Italian seasoning

1 tablespoon dried basil or ¼ cup chopped fresh basil

3 egg whites, slightly beaten

¾ cup nonfat ricotta cheese, puréed

Preheat oven to 375 degrees.

Cook noodles according to package directions. Combine chopped tomatoes, tomato sauce, tomato paste, green pepper, half of the chopped onions, the rosemary, oregano, thyme, and basil in a heavy saucepan (preferably cast-iron). Bring to a boil, stirring frequently. Simmer, covered, 10 minutes. Combine mushrooms, broccoli, red pepper, the remaining chopped onion, zucchini, and Italian seasoning in a separate container. Mix well. Mix additional basil (either chopped fresh or about a tablespoon of dried) with the slightly beaten egg whites and ricotta cheese. Spread a small amount of sauce on the bottom of a 9 x 13 baking dish. Layer on half the noodles, vegetables, sauce, and ricotta cheese mixture. Repeat. Bake 20 to 25 minutes, or until sauce is bubbling. Remove from the oven and let rest about 5 minutes before serving.

■ MACARONI AND CHEESE

1 pound macaroni

1 tablespoon flour

½ cup skim milk

1 pound nonfat Cheddar, grated or cheddar slices

Salt and pepper

Parmesan cheese, nonfat if possible, or Reggiano (a full-fat,
    full-flavored version)

Paprika

Preheat oven to 350 degrees.

Cook macaroni until tender in a medium saucepan. Combine flour and milk thoroughly and heat on medium heat. Add cheddar cheese a little at a time, stirring constantly. Season with salt and pepper. When mixture is smooth, add macaroni and pour into a nonstick casserole dish. Top with Parmesan and paprika. Bake for about 45 minutes. Serve either as a main or a side dish.

Kraft nonfat sharp cheddar slices make a very creamy sauce. They melt much better than Healthy Choice or any of the other pregrated nonfat Cheddars. If you can find Lifetime nonfat Cheddar cheese in a block, use that for the best flavor; if not, use the Kraft. Parmesan cheese has only about 1.5 grams of fat per grated tablespoon, so use an intensely flavored Parmesan like Reggiano to get maximum flavor with minimum fat or use the completely fat free so you can use as much as you desire.

■ WILD RICE

½ cup chopped onion

1 celery stalk, chopped

2 cloves garlic, peeled and minced

1 cup fresh mushrooms, chopped or sliced

½ cup chopped green onion

3 cups defatted chicken broth

1½ cups wild rice mixed with long-grain brown rice

¼ teaspoon crushed thyme

¼ teaspoon marjoram

Pinch of sage

Salt and pepper

Sauté the vegetables in a saucepan in a small amount of the broth until soft. Add the rice and sauté about 3 to 5 minutes longer. Add the remaining broth and seasonings. Bring to a boil, simmer 5 minutes, cover, turn heat to low, and cook about 50 minutes. Fluff with a fork and serve.

▪ BAKED POTATOES

Scrub the skins of russet potatoes until clean. Bake for about 50 to 60 minutes in oven preheated to 425 degrees.

EASY BAKED POTATOES

Top with picante sauce or any leftover vegetables.

LOADED BAKED POTATOES

Mix in Butter Buds, onion powder, salt, pepper, and garlic powder to taste. Top with:

Fat-free sour cream (Naturally Yours is the best I've found)
Grated fat-free Cheddar cheese
Smoked turkey breast bacon (see Note)
Chopped green onion

BARBECUE BAKED POTATOES

Top with:

Barbecue sauce
Grated fat-free Cheddar cheese
Diced onion

BROCCOLI CHEESE BAKED POTATOES

Top with:
Steamed fresh or frozen broccoli florets
Fat-free Cheddar slices

BAKED POTATO TOPPING

Mix one package of Butter Buds with 2 teaspoons of onion powder, ½ teaspoon garlic powder, 1 teaspoon dried parsley, and salt and pepper to taste. Put into a small spice jar and take with you for great potatoes out.

Note: To prepare turkey bacon, place 6 thin slices of deli smoked turkey beast (don't use maple or honey-cured) on a paper towel, leaving a little space around each slice. Microwave on high for 3 to 5 minutes or until the turkey is evenly brown. Don't overcook; it'll go from brown to black and burned in just a few seconds. Remove, and let cool before crumbling and storing.

ROASTED POTATOES

SERVES 4

½ teaspoon garlic powder

½ teaspoon onion powder

½ teaspoon pepper

1 teaspoon paprika

1 teaspoon crushed rosemary or a favorite herb or mixture of
    herbs

Salt

8 new potatoes, quartered

2 tablespoons chicken broth (approximately)

Preheat oven to 425 degrees.

Combine all the seasonings in a plastic zip bag, seal, and shake to mix well. Place quartered potatoes in bag, seal, and shake to coat. Remove potatoes and place on a foil-covered cookie sheet. Sprinkle or spritz with chicken broth. Place in preheated oven and bake for approximately 30 to 40 minutes.

■ SWEET POTATOES

4 sweet potatoes

½ cup brown sugar

1 package Butter Buds

½ jigger bourbon

Zest of 1 orange

Onion powder

½ cup freshly squeezed orange juice

Preheat oven to 450 degrees.

Bake sweet potatoes about 1 hour. Remove from skins, place in a bowl, and sprinkle with Butter Buds. Add all the other ingredients and mix well either by hand or with a mixer.

Note: You may add nutmeg, cardamom, and/or cinnamon. These spices are very strong so add just a pinch or two at a time.

■ CORNBREAD STUFFING

You'll need to make two 9-inch-square cornbreads for the stuffing. Prepare the recipe twice instead of doubling all the ingredients, but bake the two pans at the same time.

CORNBREAD

1 cup yellow cornmeal

1 cup all-purpose flour

4 teaspoons baking powder

½ teaspoon salt

¼ cup applesauce

1 cup evaporated skim milk or buttermilk

2 egg whites, slightly beaten

Preheat oven to 400 degrees.

Heat a 9 x 9 pan in oven. Combine dry ingredients. Add applesauce, milk, and beaten egg whites. Mix just until blended. Pour into hot pan. Bake 20 to 25 minutes, or until tester comes out clean.

STUFFING:

3 ribs celery, finely chopped

4 green onions, finely chopped

1 can defatted chicken broth

2 (9 x 9) cornbreads, crumbled

Pinch or two of poultry seasoning

Brown celery and onions. Place in a large bowl. Add chicken broth. Add crumbled cornbread and poultry seasoning and mix thoroughly, adding more broth if needed to reach the desired moisture level.

Variations

Add finely chopped mushrooms, finely chopped oysters, green peppers, or corn.

■ CORN CASSEROLE

1 onion, peeled and chopped

1 can chopped green chile peppers

2 "Egg Beaters" or 3 egg whites

½ pint nonfat sour cream

1 can creamed corn in liquid

1 can whole kernel corn in liquid

1 package corn muffin mix (nonfat if possible)

1 cup fat-free Cheddar cheese

Preheat oven to 250 degrees.

Combine all ingredients except cheese in a 9 x 15 pan. Bake for 30 minutes or until set. Halfway through the baking time, top with cheese.

■ GLAZED CARROTS

4 to 6 medium carrots, thinly sliced
1 tablespoon brown sugar
½ teaspoon dry mustard
½ teaspoon garlic powder
Chicken broth

Cook carrots in a small amount of water or chicken broth until crisp-tender, about 5 to 8 minutes. Drain and set aside. Combine other ingredients with a tablespoon or more of broth and cook on medium heat for a few minutes. Add carrots and toss.

■ GARLIC CARROTS

Chicken broth
4 cloves garlic, peeled and minced
4 to 6 carrots, cut in coins
1 tablespoon Butter Buds

Heat a small amount of broth in a skillet on high. After it browns, add the garlic. Brown the garlic in the broth, adding small amounts of broth as needed. When the garlic is browned, turn the heat to medium and add the carrots and enough broth or water to cover them halfway. Cover and steam for 20 minutes. Add the Butter Buds, turn the heat up, and sauté the carrots until all the liquid is evaporated.

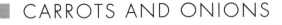

CARROTS AND ONIONS

SERVES 4

1 pound baby carrots, sliced diagonally
12 pearl onions or garlic cloves, cut in half
About 1½ cups defatted chicken broth
Salt and pepper
1 sprig each of rosemary and thyme, leaves minced

Cook the carrots and the onions or garlic in about 1 cup of broth for 15 minutes. Turn the temperature up to evaporate the broth and brown the vegetables. Season to taste with salt and pepper. Add the rosemary and thyme and cook another 15 minutes, adding a little broth at a time to prevent burning.

OLD-FASHIONED GREEN BEANS

SERVES 4

1 pound green beans
¼ teaspoon liquid smoke
1 teaspoon vinegar

Cook the green beans as you normally would, adding the seasoning ingredients.

MAPLE GREEN BEANS

SERVES 4

1 pound green beans
¼ cup maple syrup

Mix together either before or after cooking.

HONEY MUSTARD GREEN BEANS

SERVES 4

¼ cup honey
1 tablespoon mustard
1 pound green beans

Mix honey and mustard with cooked green beans.

TANGY GREEN BEANS

SERVES 4

1 pound green beans
1 teaspoon mustard
1 teaspoon sugar
1 tablespoon Butter Buds
1 teaspoon lemon juice
1 tablespoon vinegar
Salt

Cook the green beans. Combine all the remaining ingredients in a small pot. Heat on low until hot. Mix in the beans.

THAI CUCUMBER SALAD

SERVES 2 TO 4

1 Japanese or seedless cucumber

5 tablespoons sugar

½ cup white vinegar

1 teaspoon salt

3 sliced shallots or ¼ red onion, peeled and thinly sliced

½ teaspoon red chili paste or 3 fresh red chiles, seeded and
   chopped

6 to 8 sprigs cilantro

Thinly slice the cucumber and place in a nonreactive bowl. Dissolve the sugar in 1 cup boiling water. Stir in the vinegar and salt. Pour over cucumbers. Sprinkle with shallots or red onion and red chile peppers. Chill. Serve cold.

CHEESE SAUCE

MAKES ABOUT 2 CUPS

Kids, and "grown kids" will eat broccoli and cauliflower with this sauce on it. It's also great on baked potatoes.

4 garlic cloves, peeled and minced

2 tablespoons defatted chicken broth

1 can 99 percent fat-free cream of mushroom soup

8 ounces grated or sliced nonfat cheese

Sauté the garlic in a teaspoon of broth until soft. Add the soup and stir. Add the cheese, a little at a time, stirring until melted and creamy. Add skim milk to thin if necessary.

CREAM GRAVY

This is great on mashed potatoes, Chicken-Baked Steak, and Fake Fried Chicken.

    ¼ cup defatted chicken broth
    2 tablespoons quick-mixing flour
    1 cup evaporated skim milk
    ½ teaspoon onion powder

Add the chicken broth to the flour to make a thick liquid. Pour into a saucepan and slowly add the evaporated skim milk; stir in the onion powder. Bring to a boil, stirring constantly. Reduce heat and simmer at least 5 minutes.

The broth and milk ratios may be reversed for a lighter gravy.

PICO DE GALLO

SERVES 4 TO 6

This doesn't keep very well, so make it up at the last minute and make only as much as you need. You can turn it into a zesty tomato sauce by cooking it.

    2 firm, ripe tomatoes
    2 jalapeños, ribs and seeds removed
    1 small onion, peeled
    1 clove garlic, peeled
    8 sprigs cilantro
    1 tablespoon fresh lime juice
    Salt

Finely chop the tomatoes, jalapeños, onion, garlic, and cilantro. Mix, stir in lime juice, and salt to taste. Serve chilled.

PEANUT BUTTER SPREAD

Even rice cakes taste good topped with this. It's a perfect low-fat filling for sandwiches instead of the traditional peanut butter. An option for people who don't want dairy products is to use 1 cup of rinsed canned white beans instead of the ricotta cheese.

1 cup nonfat ricotta

¼ cup unhomogenized smooth peanut butter, oil poured off

2½ teaspoons vanilla

½ teaspoon cinnamon

4 teaspoons sugar, honey, or artificial sweetener

Skim milk as needed to thin

Combine in a food processor until smooth.

CHEWY BROWNIES

6 tablespoons cocoa powder

2 cups sugar

1½ cups flour

1 teaspoon baking powder

1 teaspoon salt

1 cup nonfat vanilla yogurt

1 tablespoon Karo syrup

1 teaspoon vanilla

Preheat oven to 350 degrees.

Mix the dry ingredients together. Mix wet ingredients in a separate bowl. Stir them into the cocoa mix. Bake in a 9 x 13 pan for 30 minutes.

ANY BERRIES FOOL PARFAITS

SERVES 4

½ cup blueberries or blackberries, fresh or frozen

½ cup strawberries or raspberries, fresh or frozen

1 teaspoon lemon juice

3 tablespoons sugar

1 cup evaporated skim milk, chilled in the freezer 1 hour

1 teaspoon vanilla or Grand Marnier

In a food processor purée the berries separately. Place the berries in separate small saucepans, adding ½ teaspoon lemon juice and ½ tablespoon sugar to each. Cook on medium heat until thickened—just a few minutes. Remove from heat and cool. Whip the chilled evaporated skim milk with the remaining sugar and the 2 tablespoons vanilla. Remove about a third and combine with the strawberries; do the same with the blueberries. Layer in parfait glasses, first the strawberries, then the remaining third of the whipped milk, then the blueberries. Chill in the freezer for a few hours for ice cream consistency. Garnish with additional berries and/or mint leaves.

SIMPLE FRUIT SORBET

SERVES 4

4 cups frozen fruit (strawberries, raspberries, or blueberries)

¼ cup sugar

¼ cup skim milk

2 tablespoons Grand Marnier or your favorite liqueur

Purée the berries in a food processor. Transfer to a blender, add the other ingredients, and purée again. Stir to make sure you get an even purée. Continue blending until smooth. Serve immediately.

ORANGES WITH GRAND MARNIER

If you want to impress your company with a simple dessert this is a great way to do it.

Zest of 4 oranges, all white pith removed

4 medium oranges

¾ cup sugar

½ cup Grand Marnier

If you have removed the zest with a knife, julienne the zest. (If you have used a zesting tool, you should have julienned strips.) Place the zest in a pot with just enough water to cover and bring to a boil. Discard the water, replace with fresh water, and bring to a boil again. Repeat, so the rind has been boiled 3 times with fresh water each time. Remove and discard the white pith from the oranges. Slice the oranges in ¼-inch-thick rounds, as you would for a garnish. Place the sugar and ¼ cup of water in a pot and heat on high. Let sugar melt without stirring. When it becomes dark brown, turn off the heat, add the rind, and stir to mix well. Add the Grand Marnier and another ¼ cup of water to the mixture and stir until the caramel dissolves and is of an even consistency. Add the oranges to the mixture and simmer for about 5 to 7 minutes on medium heat, stirring occasionally. Remove the orange slices and place on a deep plate. Pour the sauce with the zest over them and refrigerate for several hours before serving.

Exercise Index

Recipe Index

chicken (*cont.*)
  rice salad, 219–20
  Santa Fe, 220
chicken feathers:
  Buffalo, 206
  Jamaican, 207
  tangy Chinese, 206
classic vegetable pizza, 210
cordon bleu chicken, 214
cornbread stuffing, 242–43
corn casserole, 243
cream gravy, 248
cucumber salad, Thai, 247

desserts:
  any berries fool parfaits, 250
  chewy brownies, 249
  oranges with Grand Marnier,
    251
  simple fruit sorbet, 250
dumplings, 213
  spinach ricotta, 235

easy baked potatoes, 239

fajita marinade, homemade, 215
fajitas, quick, 215
fake fried chicken, 216
fettuccine, lemon shrimp, 223
fool parfaits, any berries, 250
fried chicken, fake, 216
fruit sorbet, simple, 250

garlic carrots, 244
gazpacho, 202
glaze, for stuffed turkey tenderloin,
    223
glazed carrots, 244
Grand Marnier, oranges with,
    251
gravy, cream, 248
green beans:
  honey mustard, 246
  maple, 246
  old-fashioned, 245
  tangy, 246

grilled lemon-lime chicken, 217
guacamole, asparagus, 204

ham and chicken jambalaya,
    218
homemade fajita marinade, 215
honey mustard green beans, 246
hummus, 205

Jamaican chicken feathers, 207
jambalaya, chicken and ham,
    218

lasagne, vegetable, 236
lemon-lime grilled chicken, 217
lemon shrimp fettuccine, 223
lime-lemon grilled chicken, 217
loaded baked potatoes, 239

macaroni and cheese, 237
maple green beans, 246
marinades:
  homemade fajita, 215
  for shrimp scampi, 225
  variations, for chicken feathers,
    206–7
meatloaf, most requested, 230
Mexican pizza, 209
middle eastern pizza, 210
most requested meatloaf, 230
muffins:
  apple oat, 198
  breakfast on the run, 196
  power, 195
mushroom risotto, 234
mustard:
  honey green beans, 246
  sauce, pork with, 233

oat apple muffins, 198
old-fashioned green beans, 245
omelets, 199
onions and carrots, 245
oranges with Grand Marnier,
    251
oriental pizza, 209